BACK PAIN

Questions you have . . . Answers you need

Other Books From The People's Medical Society

Take This Book to the Hospital With You

How to Evaluate and Select a Nursing Home

Medicine on Trial

Medicare Made Easy

Your Medical Rights

Getting the Most for Your Medical Dollar

Take This Book to the Gynecologist With You

Take This Book to the Obstetrician With You

Blood Pressure: Questions You Have . . . Answers You Need

Your Heart: Questions You Have . . . Answers You Need

The Consumer's Guide to Medical Lingo

150 Ways to Be a Savvy Medical Consumer

Take This Book to the Pediatrician With You

100 Ways to Live to 100

Dial 800 for Health

Your Complete Medical Record

Arthritis: Questions You Have . . . Answers You Need

Diabetes: Questions You Have . . . Answers You Need

Prostate: Questions You Have . . . Answers You Need

Vitamins and Minerals: Questions You Have . . . Answers You Need

Good Operations—Bad Operations

The Complete Book of Relaxation Techniques

Test Yourself for Maximum Health

Misdiagnosis: Woman As a Disease

Yoga Made Easy

Massage Made Easy

Hearing Loss: Questions You Have . . . Answers You Need

Asthma: Questions You Have . . . Answers You Need

Depression: Questions You Have . . . Answers You Need

BACK PAIN

Questions you have ...Answers you need

By Sandra Salmans

People's Medical Society
Allentown, Pennsylvania

The People's Medical Society is a nonprofit consumer health organization dedicated to the principles of better, more responsive and less expensive medical care. Organized in 1983, the People's Medical Society puts previously unavailable medical information into the hands of consumers so that they can make informed decisions about their own health care.

Membership in the People's Medical Society is $20 a year and includes a subscription to the *People's Medical Society Newsletter*. For information, write to the People's Medical Society, 462 Walnut Street, Allentown, PA 18102, or call 610-770-1670.

This and other People's Medical Society publications are available for quantity purchase at discount. Contact the People's Medical Society for details.

Printed in the United States of America

Library of Congress Cataloging-in-Publication Data

Salmans, Sandra.

Back pain : questions you have, answers you need / by Sandra Salmans.

p. cm.

Includes bibliographical references and index.

ISBN 1-882606-19-1 (trade paper)

1. Backache—Popular works. I. Title.

RD771.B217S25 1995

617.5'64—dc20 95-5937

CIP

4 5 6 7 8 9 0

First printing, March 1995

CONTENTS

INTRODUCTION

Everyone has a back-pain story. I once threw my back out simply reaching to open the front door. That incident cost me two days' work, about $100 in doctor visits and medications, and at least two weeks of constant pain. Yet that was not a very serious incident. There are millions of people, every day, suffering very serious problems that cause excruciating back pain.

The prevalence of back pain and the many reasons it occurs has made the condition an industry in America. There are physicians who limit their practices to back pain. There are back-pain clinics. There are pills, salves, exercises, and machinery made or designed to alleviate or prevent pains in your back. And back surgeries are some of the most frequently performed operations. Chiropractors treat back pain. Massage therapists offer treatment. Physical therapists and exercise specialists have regimens designed to both eliminate or reduce pain, and possibly even prevent it.

On the one hand, all this attention to back pain has propelled our knowledge of why it occurs and how to treat it to new levels. On the other hand, the fact that the "industry" has little oversight and regulation makes it rife for charlatans or pseudo-professionals to con or dupe an unsuspecting public with offers of relief and cure that have little or no basis in fact.

That is why we offer *Back Pain: Questions You Have . . . Answers You Need.* Our goal is to help you find relief for the pain you or a loved one is suffering. The information you will read in this book comes directly from the medical literature. We have researched and examined the studies, talked with the experts and reviewed the bona fide medical reports to present the most unbiased information available on why back pain occurs and what you can do about it.

Like the other books in our *Questions You Have . . . Answers You Need* series, *Back Pain: Questions You Have . . . Answers You Need* is presented in an easy-to-follow, understandable format. This format has been hailed by the hundreds of thousands of readers of our other books as offering the most comprehensive discussion of the subject in an uncomplicated way.

As the nation's largest, nonprofit, consumer health advocacy organization, the People's Medical Society is dedicated to providing you with the most useful medical and health information available. We feel that we have again accomplished that goal in this book.

Charles B. Inlander
President
People's Medical Society

BACK PAIN

**Questions
you
have
. . . Answers
you
need**

Terms printed in boldface can be found in the glossary, beginning on page 163. Only the first mention of the word in the text will be boldfaced.

We have tried to use male and female pronouns in an egalitarian manner throughout the book. Any imbalance in usage has been in the interest of readability.

1 THE BACK, UP FRONT

Q: Where does back pain come from?

A: Unfortunately, not even the experts can tell you that. (And if someone tries, well, watch your back!) The back is one of the most intricate biomechanical parts of our anatomy, and the sources of back pain are among the most elusive. A widely quoted figure is that 85 percent of back pain is **idiopathic**—medical language for "we don't know the cause."

What we do know is that back pain appears to come from a number of different sources, and that it seems to be triggered by a vast range of events, from reaching too high for a tennis ball to bending over to pick up a straight pin. It depends on the event, the individual and, ultimately, the back.

Q: Sounds like I need to know more about the back. How does it work?

A: A crash course in the "mechanics" of the back would be a good idea before we go on in Chapters 2 and 3 to discuss how backs go bad.

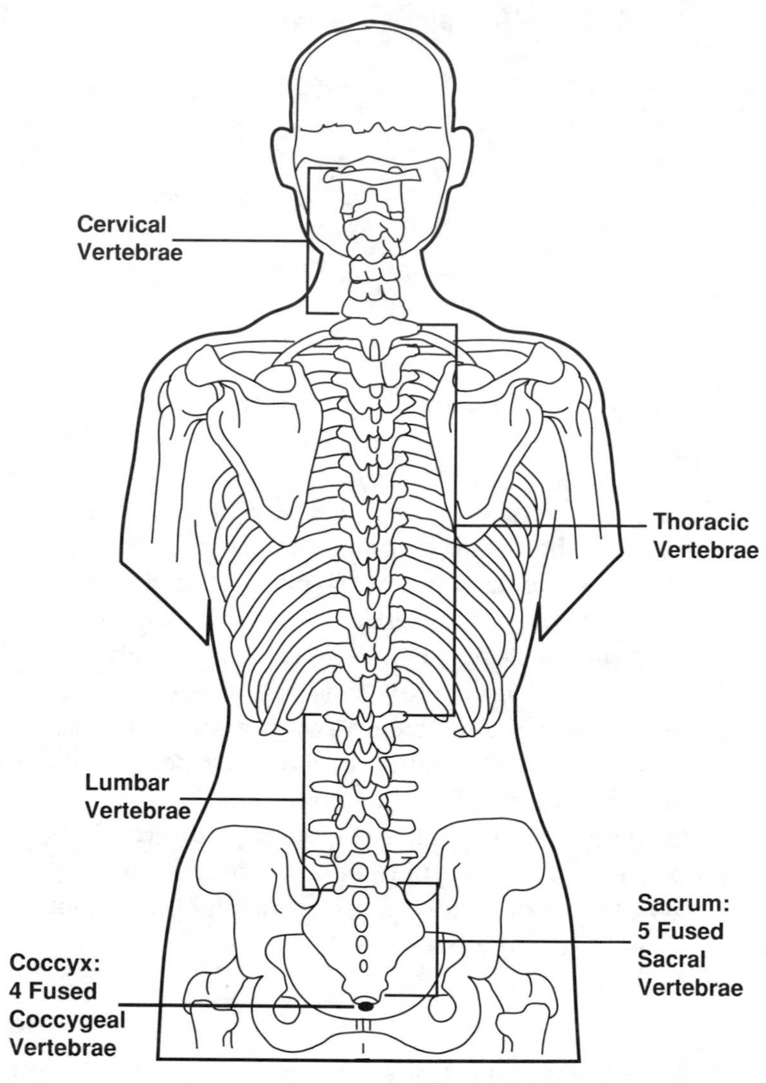

THE HUMAN SPINE

Let's start with the **spinal column**, which is comprised of 24—or 33, depending on how you count them—**vertebrae**. Each vertebra is cylindrical and about an inch high.

The upper portion, consisting of seven vertebrae beginning at the base of the skull, is the neck or **cervical spine**. The midportion is the midback or **thoracic spine**, consisting of 12 vertebrae which are enclosed by the rib cage. The lower region, from below the ribs to the hips, is the **lumbar spine** or the low back—five vertebrae that are the heftiest of the 24.

Q: That adds up to 24. What happened to the other nine?

A: Everyone is born with 33 vertebrae, but the extra nine, at the base of the spine, usually grow together by adulthood. Below the lowest lumbar, five vertebrae fuse together to form the triangular bone called the **sacrum**. The joint where the sacrum joins the hipbones is the **sacroiliac**, which at one time was blamed, unfairly, for most back pain. Remember "my aching sacroiliac"?

Finally, four tiny bones fuse together to create a tail-like appendage called the **coccyx**, or tailbone.

Q: I've heard doctors use phrases like L1 and T3 when they discuss the back. What are they talking about?

A: For medical purposes, there's a sequential letter and number system for the vertebrae. The letter is taken from the region where the vertebra is located, and the number from its position in that region, top to bottom. Hence labels like L1 (the first vertebra in the lumbar spine) and T3 (the third vertebra in the thoracic region).

Q: Are the vertebrae those knobs I feel down the middle of my back?

A: No, those are projections called **spinous processes**. Stacked on top of each other, the vertebrae form a hollow tube called the **spinal canal**. The spinous processes overlap each other slightly to form an extra protective wrapping around the spinal canal.

Q: Is that all there is to the backbone?

A: There's lots more. Between each pair of vertebrae is one of those **discs** you've probably heard a lot about. The disc is a flat, round structure, about a half-inch thick, consisting of an **annulus**, or tough outer ring of **collagen**, encircling a gelatinous nucleus, or center, consisting mostly of water. The disc is often described as a jelly doughnut in the back.

The 23 discs account for about one-third the length of your spine. They're the largest organs in your body without their own blood supply. When they're young and healthy, discs absorb a lot of water—so much so that you grow taller in the night, as your discs swell, and lose a fraction of an inch during the course of the day, as your discs compress.

Q: What purpose do discs serve?

A: Apart from separating the vertebrae, they act as the spine's cushions or shock absorbers. They compress when weight is put on them, and spring back when it's removed.

Q: What holds it all together?

A: Keeping the spine aligned and playing a critical role in the way it functions, are the paired joints that connect the vertebrae, known as **facet joints**; and the soft tissues—nerves, muscles, **ligaments**, tendons (which connect muscle to bone) and cartilage.

Q: Let's start with the facet joints. Where are they?

A: They're extensions at the rear of each vertebra. They act as hinges between the vertebrae, connecting each to the one below it, and guiding, directing and controlling the movement of the spine. Together with soft tissues, they're the reason that backs rarely "go out," as people say they do.

Part of the facets' lining is composed of **synovial** tissue, which nourishes and lubricates the joints, letting them move smoothly and without friction. As we'll see in Chapter 2, however, this is also a source of trouble.

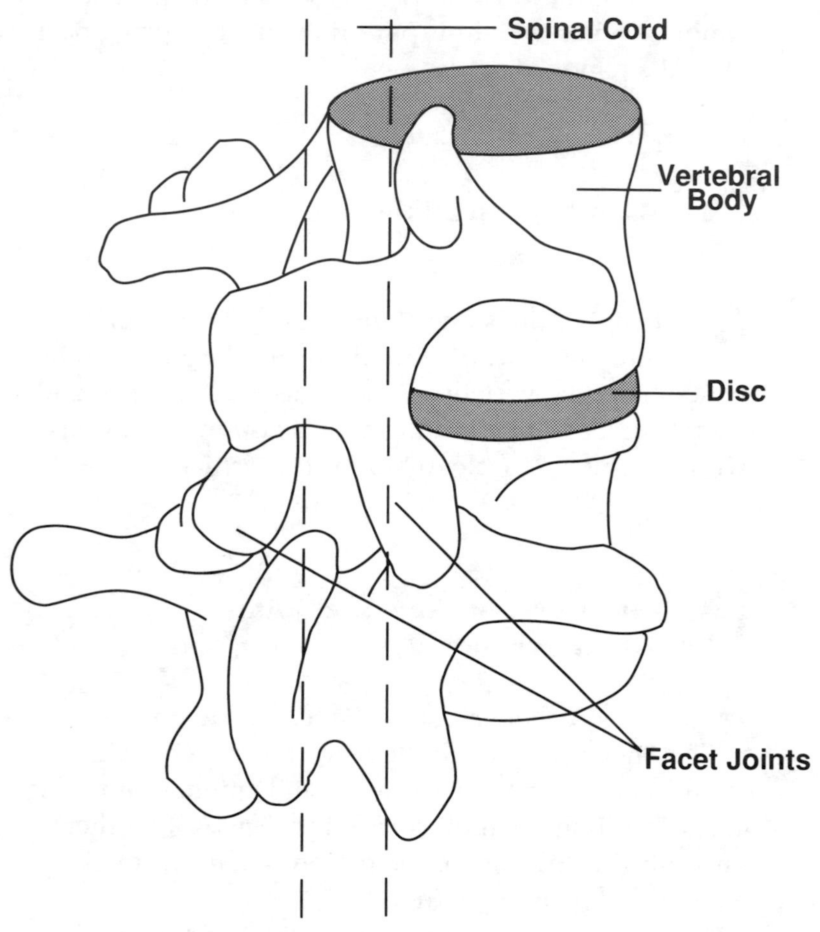

THE VERTEBRAL JOINTS, REAR VIEW

Q: Where are the nerves?

A: Nerves—31 pairs in all—branch off from the **spinal cord**, which is inside the spinal canal. The spinal cord is an extension of the brain that ends at the top of the lumbar spine. When you bend your neck forward, the whole spinal cord moves upward in the spinal canal.

The spinal cord carries impulses through nerves from the brain to the rest of the body and, in reverse, conveys information from the body to the brain. At L1, the cord ends in an important bundle of nerves which, because it's long and stringy, is called the **cauda equina** (Latin for "horse's tail").

Through the nerve exits, known as **foramen**, each section of the spine governs, in a sense, specific sections of the body: the cervical vertebrae for the arms and hands, the thoracic vertebrae for the torso, and the lumbar vertebrae for the lower limbs.

Q: And muscles? What do they do?

A: There are two main muscle groups—a total of 140 muscles—that protect the back: **extensors** and **flexors**. The extensors, also known as the **erector spinae** muscles (because they hold your spine erect), attach to the back part of the spine and pass from one vertebra to another, although each individual extensor spans only two or three vertebrae. These are the muscles that allow us to straighten up and lift things.

Flexor muscles are in the front and include all the abdominal muscles. They allow us to bend forward, but they're also important during lifting because some of them—the obliques—help control the amount of **lordosis**, the natural curve in the low back.

There's also a third important group consisting of the **psoas** muscles, whose main job is to move the legs. They begin at the front of the lumbar spine and go across the hip joint to the thighbone.

All these muscles are covered by a fibrous tissue called **fascia**.

Q: You mentioned ligaments, too. What do they do?

A: Ligaments, which are strong bands of fibrous tissue, help hold it all together. Each vertebra is connected to the next by several ligaments, whose elasticity allows a certain amount of motion.

INCIDENCE AND RISK GROUPS

Q: Okay, so much for mechanics' school. How common is back pain?

A: It's extremely common. Alf L. Nachemson, M.D., an **orthopedic surgeon** and prominent researcher at the University of Göteborg, Sweden, has estimated that "sometime during our active lives 80 percent of us will experience back pain to some extent."

National statistics indicate that 15 to 20 percent of the U.S. population has low-back problems during any given year, and that figure rises to 50 percent of working-age people. According to the National Center for Health Statistics, back pain ranks second only to cold symptoms as a reason people give for seeing a doctor. And in 1988, low-back problems were the seventh leading reason for all hospitalizations in the United States.

Q: What's the cost of back pain, on a national basis?

A: As you might expect from those statistics, back pain is a sizable component of the nation's health-care bill. According to a study by The Travelers Companies, a nationwide insurer, bad backs cost U.S. businesses $30 billion a year in lost time and medical benefits.

If you're wondering why we're using a figure furnished by an insurance company rather than, say, by the National Institutes of Health, it's because insurers pay huge bills for disability from bad backs. Among occupation-related injuries, low-back pain is the major cause of disability in young patients; in people over 45 years of age, it's the third leading cause, after cardiac and arthritic conditions.

Q: You've been talking generally about the back. Is there a particular area where pain occurs?

A: While back pain can occur anywhere in the spine, usually it occurs in the lumbar spine, or low back. A distant second is the cervical spine, or neck.

Q: Why does back pain usually occur in the low back?

A: The low back is subjected to more stress and strain than any other section of the spine. Just standing erect focuses about 100 pounds of pressure on the lumbar area; sitting increases those forces by almost 50 percent. Lifting puts even more pressure on the low back.

Since the low back bears so much of the weight, discs there are more subject to rupture and muscles to tear than elsewhere in the spinal column. By contrast, because they're fairly rigid, thoracic vertebrae don't permit much movement, and thus aren't injured as often as the other vertebrae.

Q: Who gets low-back pain?

A: Back pain is an equal-opportunity affliction: Men and women of all races are affected equally. However, there are a number of other factors, notably age, heredity and occupation, that affect the odds you'll develop back pain. We'll discuss the role of age and heredity in specific back problems in Chapters 2 and 3.

For the moment, however, we'll note that people who are physically unfit—not disabled, just out of shape—are at relatively high risk for back problems. Norbert Sander, M.D., the director and founder of the Preventive and Sports Medicine Center in Manhattan, told the *New York Times* that more than 90 percent of the cases of low-back pain he sees are the result of muscular problems caused by lack of exercise, weak muscles or overweight.

Q: But aren't there types of work that are particularly likely to lead to back pain?

A: There's a broad spectrum of jobs in which back problems tend to develop. Some are predictable: People who perform heavy manual labor or drive a motor vehicle all day—occupations that subject the spine to constant vibration—report a high incidence of back pain. On the other hand, one study found that white-collar professionals account for 28 percent of patients with **chronic** back pain—that is, pain lasting for more than two or three months.

Gunnar Anderson, a leading Swedish back researcher, has listed the occupational dangers as follows:

- physically heavy work
- static work postures
- frequent bending and twisting
- lifting and forceful movements
- repetitive work (such as assembly-line jobs)
- vibrations

Q: What about body build? Do tall people get backaches more often than short people?

A: It's not clear. A number of widely held beliefs about bad backs and body types are being challenged by researchers. Most studies indicate there's no strong correlation between body build and back pain. However, some research does suggest that people who are tall are more likely to develop bad backs. And within the medical community there's a general consensus that an individual who is obese has higher odds of developing a bad back.

Q: How does obesity lead to back pain?

A: A large belly shifts the center of gravity forward, making the erector muscles work harder and exert greater force to keep the spine erect. This puts more pressure on the spine at both the facet joints and the discs.

The same applies for pregnant women, but their problems are magnified by the production, in the later stages of pregnancy, of a hormone called relaxin. This hormone relaxes the ligaments in the pelvis, to ease delivery, but it also relaxes ligaments in the lumbar spine, undermining the back's strength.

Q: I'd always heard that bad posture will give you a bad back. Is that true?

A: That's another widely held belief that's being challenged. Many studies indicate there's no connection between "voluntary" moderately poor posture and a bad back. However, extremely bad posture—which is generally involuntary—that leads to a permanent spinal curvature can indeed cause back pain, as we discuss in Chapter 3.

Q: What about leg-length differences? Do they cause back pain?

A: Although there's some professional disagreement on this issue, the majority of discrepancies in leg length are also being discounted as a factor. According to Augustus A. White III, M.D., a professor of orthopedic surgery at Harvard Medical School and author of *Your Aching Back,* differences as great as three-fourths of an inch are "inconsequential."

Q: Is it true that very large breasts can cause back pain?

A: Yes, for a couple of reasons. Just like a large belly, extremely large breasts shift the center of gravity and put additional strain on the muscles of the low back. Furthermore, women who are self-conscious about the size of their breasts may try to minimize them by rolling their shoulders inward and rounding their thoracic spine. All told, they can develop neck strain and low-back pain.

Q: Are there any other risk groups?

A: A great many people may be more susceptible to back pain because of **psychosocial** rather than physical factors. Various studies indicate that such factors as stress, living alone and satisfaction with one's work and/or life can have an impact on the health of one's back.

Chapter 2 discusses connections between some specific back problems and stress.

Q: You mean people who don't like their jobs get bad backs?

A: Yes, or perhaps they're more likely to complain about the pain. A study by the Spine Resource Clinic at the University of Washington, in Seattle, of 31,200 employees at the Boeing Company found that workers who said they "hardly ever" enjoyed their job tasks were 2½ times more likely to report a back injury than those who "almost always" enjoyed their work.

The Boeing study found a higher incidence of back problems in workers who had had negative job evaluations within the previous six months. Personality conflicts with the boss also seemed to have a direct correlation with back pain. "The job itself does not seem to matter as much as how well you get along with your supervisor," said Stanley J. Bigos, M.D., an orthopedic surgeon who is founder and director of the clinic.

Q: What's the outlook for recovering from back pain?

A: Excellent. Most people with **acute** back pain—that is, pain that's come on suddenly—recover on their own. According to Stephen Hochschuler, M.D., cofounder of the Texas Back Institute, in Plano, within two or three weeks 70 percent of people get better, and by 12 weeks, 80 percent feel better.

Of the relatively small minority who seek medical care, the vast majority recover after their visits, and only 10 percent or less have residual pain two months after the initial episode.

Q: In that case, why doesn't everybody recover quickly?

A: There are a number of factors. Some conditions, as we'll discuss in Chapters 2 and 3, are extremely difficult or even impossible to treat; in certain cases, the pain may even be preferable to the treatment. Complicating the treatment issue is that back problems are often quite difficult to diagnose; if and when treatment doesn't work, it's accordingly difficult to determine why.

At the same time, there's evidence that more extraneous factors, including psychosocial factors and the anticipation of compensation for back pain, may significantly impede recovery.

Q: What's the prognosis for people with chronic back pain?

A: Comparatively, quite bleak. The odds of returning to work for these people diminish sharply over time, and become minuscule if the pain persists for 24 months, according to a Swedish study. An estimated 8 to 10 percent of patients with chronic low-back pain eventually become physically and/or emotionally disabled, according to C. David Tollison, Ph.D., of the Center for Health and Occupational Services at the Greenville Hospital System, in Greenville, South Carolina.

Q: Emotionally disabled, too? So people with back pain develop other problems?

A: Depression is a common syndrome in people with chronic pain, and that includes chronic back pain. According to the *British Medical Journal,* a recent survey of patients seen in 10 outpatient clinics in Britain found that nearly half of those with chronic back pain had a psychological component to their pain.

Admittedly, the precise cause-and-effect relationship of back pain and depression is unclear and, as we indicated earlier, people who are unhappy seem more likely to develop back problems. However, research by J. Hampton Atkinson, M.D., a psychiatrist at the School of Medicine, University of California-San Diego, in La Jolla, and others found that in the great majority of cases the first episode of depression occurred *after* pain onset. When compared with controls, the research subjects didn't have a higher-than-average risk of mood disorder before the pain began, according to the article published in the *Journal of Psychosomatic Medicine* in 1994.

Q: Do they develop other physical ailments?

A: Yes. In the medical community, people with chronic low-back pain are often described as "somatizers" because they tend to report multiple **somatic** complaints beyond back pain itself. In a review of research in this area, Atkinson notes that as many as 75 percent of chronic back patients report "numerous bodily complaints" aside from pain. The more severe those complaints, furthermore, the likelier the person was to have drinking problems.

Other research has found that people with chronic back pain often tend to develop headaches that begin or worsen markedly after the onset of back pain. The headaches are particularly severe for women with chronic back pain, who are three times likelier to have migraines than women without it.

Q: Why would chronic back-pain sufferers get more migraines?

A: The researchers, from the Division of Behavioral Medicine at the St. Louis University Health Sciences Center, in St. Louis, Missouri, proposed a number of theories. They speculated that the headaches had a physiological source; to minimize the pain, people may overuse and underuse certain muscles, sometimes at sites remote from the original pain, and thus bring on migraines.

Psychosocial factors—specifically, depression—were another explanation. Finally, the researchers suggested that the overuse of painkillers to relieve low-back pain might contribute to migraine.

Q: Earlier you mentioned that recovery might be affected by compensation. You mean whether people get paid for their pain?

A: That's right. In 1990, back injuries accounted for 22 percent of all workers' compensation claims and 31 percent of all payments, according to the National Safety Council. And that's not counting all the people in car accidents who sue for damages related to **whiplash** or other spinal injury.

Various studies have shown that people seeking compensation are slower to recover than those who aren't. For example, a study by Tollison, published in the *Southern Medical Journal* in 1993, found that "compensation patients" took more medicine, rated their pain as significantly greater and were slower to return to work than their noncompensation counterparts.

Q: Does that mean that people exaggerate their pain in order to collect?

A: That's the obvious conclusion, and Tollison's study is the only one to reach it. Of course, it's also possible that the people in line to collect are slower to heal because they're more severely injured than the average.

Given the nature of back pain, it's impossible to say which conclusion is correct. However, we'll note that many **orthopedists** routinely suspect fraud or exaggeration when they treat people in litigation. "The presence of pending legal action is a tip-off to most of us that the patient may be using symptoms to obtain money or to avoid responsibilities," Burton Sack, M.D., of Boston University, wrote in *Modern Medicine* in 1992. "It is almost impossible for this individual to get well during litigation."

Q: What about recurrence?

A: Studies indicate that, once you've had back pain, your likelihood of having it again increases fourfold. According to Augustus White of Harvard, statistics show that about 60 percent of patients with acute, incapacitating low-back pain are likely to have another attack within two years.

That's why prevention, discussed in Chapter 5, is so important.

HEALTH-CARE PROFESSIONALS

Q: Who would I see for back problems?

A: Nearly half of people with back pain who choose to consult a doctor are treated by their primary-care physician or internist. About one-third consult orthopedists or orthopedic surgeons, medical doctors (M.D.'s) who have been trained specifically in the diagnosis and treatment of the musculoskeletal system. Because of their training, it's orthopedists who perform most back surgery.

It's worth noting that there's specialization even within orthopedics, with some doctors concentrating on the neck and shoulders or on the low back. Extremely complicated back operations may be best left in the hands of a specially trained spine surgeon.

Quite a few back-pain sufferers see an **osteopath**. A doctor of osteopathy (D.O.) is a fully licensed physician who has received a medical education and postgraduate training similar to that of an M.D., and can also prescribe drugs.

However, osteopathic training emphasizes the musculoskeletal system—the body's bones, joints, ligaments, tendons and muscles—and holds that imbalances and abnormalities in that system can affect the way we function generally. One of the techniques osteopaths use is **spinal manipulation**.

Q: Are there other physicians who specialize in back problems?

A: Because back pain has so many causes, a number of other types of physicians—M.D.'s or D.O.'s—have a special interest in the back.

Physiatrists have been trained specifically in physical medicine and rehabilitation—diagnosing and treating patients with impairments or disabilities that involve the musculoskeletal, nervous and other systems. Unlike orthopedists and osteopaths, they're not licensed to perform surgery, and they emphasize noninvasive treatment such as **physical therapy**, lifestyle changes and many other therapies.

Rheumatologists specialize in treating diseases of the joints, muscles, bones and tendons. They've undergone special training in diagnosing and treating various types of **arthritis** and other rheumatic diseases, which often affect the back and cause pain.

Neurosurgeons and **neurologists** focus on the brain, spinal cord and peripheral nerves of the body. They often deal with injuries to the brain or spinal cord resulting from trauma or tumors. Neurologists diagnose and treat disorders; neurosurgeons perform surgery.

Q: Aside from M.D.'s and D.O.'s, what other health-care professionals treat bad backs?

A: A number of other health-care professionals specialize in orthopedics. The most important—in terms of the numbers of patients they treat—are **chiropractors**. According to Paul Shekelle, M.D., a researcher at Rand in Santa Monica, California, chiropractors account for twice the number of visits for back pain as physicians. In an eight-year nationwide study, Shekelle found that 7.5 percent of the population had made at least one visit to a chiropractor, mostly for spinal problems.

Q: What is a chiropractor, exactly?

A: A doctor of **chiropractic** (D.C.) has received extensive training specifically in the musculoskeletal system. During four years at a chiropractic college, she has studied anatomy, physiology, neurophysiology, biomechanics and kinesiology.

Chiropractors cannot prescribe drugs or perform surgery. The primary treatment they offer is spinal manipulation or, as they call it, manual spinal adjustment.

The most traditional chiropractors restrict their practice to spinal manipulation. However, the ranks of the "straights," as they're called, are declining, and increasingly chiropractors are "mixers" who believe that other techniques, such as physical therapy, diet and exercise, can be helpful in treating back pain.

Q: What is spinal manipulation?

A: Using their hands, practitioners apply pressure to the spine in a specific direction and location. They maintain that this force helps restore the alignment and mobility of the vertebrae. While manipulation encompasses many different techniques, two methods are used most often:

• a nonspecific long-lever manipulation, in which parts of the body, such as arms and legs, are used as long levers to move a joint beyond its active limit of motion; and

• a specific short-level, high-velocity manipulation, in which a series of short, quick and highly controlled thrusts are applied to the back and neck.

As a technique, spinal manipulation has been practiced for centuries. In the last 50 years, however, its use has been equated with chiropractic and, partly because of this, orthopedists have considered it an ''alternative'' treatment. But that view is changing, particularly as growing numbers of people with musculoskeletal problems flock to osteopaths and chiropractors.

Q: What's the difference between the ways chiropractors and osteopaths perform spinal manipulation?

A: The short-level, high-velocity manipulation is most closely identified with chiropractors, although they use the long-lever manipulations, too. That aside, the main difference is the emphasis chiropractors place on manipulation to the exclusion of other treatments. According to one study, chiropractors delivered 94 percent of all the manipulative care for which reimbursement was sought, while osteopaths delivered 4 percent, and general practitioners and orthopedic surgeons accounted for the rest.

Q: Aren't chiropractors called "back crackers"?

A: Colloquially. The reason presumably is that, when the spine is manipulated or adjusted, there's a popping or cracking sound. The manipulation forces the surfaces of the facet joints apart, creating and then releasing a small vacuum, which creates the popping sound. It's the same sound you make when you crack your knuckles.

While many people who visit chiropractors regularly wait for their "snap, crackle and pop," the sound isn't that meaningful. It also doesn't necessarily signify that the appropriate adjustment has been made. And by the same token, if there's no noise, that doesn't mean there's been no improvement.

Q: Is spinal manipulation safe?

A: Chiropractic has an extremely good safety record, particularly for lumbar spinal manipulation; the risk for cervical spine complications is slightly higher, according to Shekelle. There have been cases where manipulation has resulted in acute disc herniation or even permanent neurological problems, including paralysis. But, given the number of people treated by chiropractors, such reports are remarkably few.

Nonetheless, there are certain individuals for whom spinal manipulation would be patently unsafe: people with fracture or disease, women in late pregnancy, or people whose pain increases with manipulation. The general consensus is that, if you have neurological symptoms such as shooting pains or numbness in the legs, you should see a physician, not a chiropractor.

Q: Isn't chiropractic controversial?

A: That depends partly on the specific chiropractor and partly on the perspective of which member of the medical establishment you're consulting. But it's fair to say that, for a growing percentage of the lay public and even the medical community, it's increasingly mainstream.

Not too long ago, the official policy of the American Medical Association (AMA) was that chiropractic was quackery; the AMA said it was unethical for doctors to associate with chiropractors. In 1987, however, after a much-publicized antitrust lawsuit in which chiropractors charged the AMA with conspiracy to monopolize medicine, the AMA was forced to recant.

These days some hospitals and health maintenance organizations embrace chiropractors. However, some orthopedists and other physicians remain highly skeptical of chiropractors' effectiveness.

Q: Why are chiropractors so controversial?

A: Apart from the fact that they compete with the medical and osteopathic establishment for the same market, one reason is chiropractors' theory that spinal adjustment corrects **subluxations**, or slight dislocations or misalignments of the vertebrae that, they maintain, irritate nerve roots and blood vessels and cause pain. Chiropractors say subluxations may be caused by just about anything: a fall, injury, an inherited spinal weakness, improper sleeping habits, poor posture, occupational hazards, obesity, stress. They maintain that subluxations are present even when they can't be seen on X-rays. But orthopedists say, if it can't be seen, it isn't there. And, whatever clinical studies show, there's no scientific proof that spinal manipulation works.

A related bone of contention is the importance chiropractic has traditionally placed on subluxations. Chiropractic practitioners, particularly the straights, maintain that subluxations can be the cause of any number of health problems—not just back pain—and that spinal adjustment can be the cure.

Q: Does adjustment help ease back pain?

A: Opinion is sharply divided on that point, but there's a growing consensus that it helps provide at least short-term relief. Chapter 2 discusses research comparing spinal manipulation with other treatments.

Q: What other non-M.D. professionals treat bad backs?

A: **Physical therapists** help patients learn exercises to improve joint and spine mobility and strengthen the muscles that hold the spine in place. They use various manipulative techniques and exercise equipment, as well as whirlpool baths, heat or cold, and massage.

Kinesiotherapists take an approach similar to that of the physical therapists, but they tend to work primarily with people needing long-term rehabilitation.

Occupational therapists' main purpose is to make you as functional as possible with your bad back. They can show you how to protect your back and carry on the normal activities of life in the best ways possible.

All three of these specialties require a bachelor's degree from an approved program. They work under a physician's direction, and with other health-care personnel as part of a team.

Q: Where would I go for treatment by one of those people?

A: Many of them are on the staff of hospitals or **back schools**. The back school—of which there are well over 1,000 in the United States, including most major cities—is an institution you may also want to consider if you have chronic or recurring back pain.

Q: What's a back school?

A: Back schools are places that teach people how to go about their daily activities while protecting their backs. They provide instruction in the mechanics of the back and what causes back pain.

While they may teach you pain-control techniques, back schools aren't pain clinics—they're much more interested in taking a "proactive" approach to a bad back. Instructors provide training in posture and movement; sometimes they even make an **ergonomic** evaluation of your workplace and the sports you play, to ensure that you're using your back in the healthiest possible way.

Q: Are they legitimate?

A: That depends on the back school, but as an institution they're generally well-regarded by the medical community (although not by insurers—reimbursement is iffy). Back schools were pioneered in Sweden at the Volvo automobile factory in the late 1960s, among other places, and today they're often found in workplaces as well as other establishments. Some are affiliated with hospitals, others are run by orthopedic surgeons, and still others by nonprofit institutions like the YMCA.

Programs range from several hours to several days or even weeks, and prices vary accordingly. Of course, some are better than others, and there are no national guidelines or standards for back schools.

You can locate them in your telephone directory or ask the orthopedist or physical therapist who's treating you.

Q: Are there "alternative" options?

A: Yes, and people with chronic back pain often seek them out to replace or supplement traditional approaches that aren't working. In addition to chiropractic—which is still considered "alternative" by the medical establishment—we'd put **massage** therapy and **acupuncture** at the top of the list of such options.

In Chapter 2, we'll discuss the effectiveness of these practices. Suffice it to note here that, if you're seeking a practitioner, beware: They're closely regulated in some states and less so in others.

Q: How do I know what kind of doctor (or other health-care practitioner) is best for me?

A: If you're like most people, you'll probably start with your primary-care doctor. There are advantages to seeing a generalist: A more specialized physician may not consider all the possible causes of back pain, including diseases or conditions that actually have nothing to do with the back.

Of course, you may not have a family doctor. And even if you do, you may end up seeing a specialist like an orthopedic surgeon or a chiropractor. If your physician can't or won't provide a referral, you can get some names of orthopedists from the North American Spine Society at (708) 698-1630. (You should be aware, however, that you'll get only the names of members of the society, which is under the same administrative umbrella as the American Academy of Orthopaedic Surgeons.)

The International Chiropractors Association will give you the names only of their members; try your local telephone directory for wider listings.

DIAGNOSING BACK PAIN

Q: How is back pain diagnosed?

A: The first thing most practitioners do—whether they're medical doctors, osteopaths or chiropractors—is take a history to try to determine what triggered the pain. Then they conduct a physical examination to help determine the extent of your mobility, whether the pain comes from muscles, discs, nerves or other sources, and what part of the back is involved.

For a start, you're asked to stand and walk. Probably you'll have to bend forward, backward and sideways, to twist in various directions, and to walk on your heels and then on your toes.

The practitioner feels your spine for areas of heat, swelling, nodules or tenderness, and palpates your back for painful muscle knots. He tests the strength of each muscle group, and may even measure the circumference of each thigh and calf to see if there's been any muscle atrophy, which could indicate a disc problem.

He may also check your **Babinski reflex** by stroking the bottom of your foot. If your toes curl down, that indicates there's no damage to the spinal cord or brain.

Q: What about those little rubber hammers doctors have? Don't they test reflexes?

A: Yes. When a practitioner taps your knee or elbow with his hammer, he's checking your reflexes to determine whether there's nerve damage. If the nerve is compressed, the muscle contraction may be weak and the reflex slow and poor.

Q: Are there any specific tests for neck or low-back pain?

A: If the practitioner suspects cervical spine problems, she may test neck flexion by having you perform certain movements such as trying to touch your ear to your shoulder. Possibly she'll test sensation in your fingers, alternating hands, while you indicate whether the touch feels normal on both sides.

On the other hand, if low-back pain seems to be the problem, you'll have to take the straight-leg-raising test, in which you lie or sit on an examining table and raise each leg to see how far it can go before the pain becomes severe. This helps determine whether spinal nerves are involved.

Q: What about other diagnostic tests and measurements?

A: That depends on what kind of practitioner is treating you. According to a recent study conducted at the University of Washington, the Group Health Cooperative of Puget Sound, and the Seattle Veterans Affairs Medical Center, in Seattle, Washington, there's little consensus among the medical specialties on which tests should be ordered for three common types of low-back pain. Even within specialties, the physicians were often divided about the value of specific tests.

Q: Since they're interested in the backbone, don't they use X-rays?

A: "Plain films," as doctors call conventional X-rays, have increasingly fallen out of favor with orthopedists because they're too insensitive to identify the causes of most chronic pain. While they provide good detail of bone, they don't reveal much about changes in soft tissue such as muscle and ligament.

And in disc disease and other chronic conditions, at least half of the bony tissue needs to be destroyed before X-rays disclose any sign of deterioration, according to Robert D. Crane, M.D., a radiologist at the Virginia Mason Medical Center, in Seattle, Washington.

Q: Then X-rays shouldn't be taken at all?

A: Because they do offer a good picture of bone, experts say, X-rays still have a major role when the back pain may be due to trauma or fracture. And, whatever the arguments against them, some practitioners —including many chiropractors—still order X-rays on the initial visit.

Q: Are there other imaging techniques that are more effective in making a diagnosis?

A: Yes. **CT (computerized axial tomographic) scans** are superior to X-rays, and **magnetic resonance imaging (MRI)** is better than CT scans. The main drawback is that both are expensive—the MRI prohibitively so, if you're paying for it yourself.

Still other diagnostic imaging techniques have been developed specifically for back problems. These include **discography** and **myelography**, both of which are used to visualize disc problems. We describe both procedures in Chapter 2. Suffice it to say for now that neither procedure is foolproof and both can be quite painful. These tests and others might be ordered by orthopedists and osteopaths.

Q: Is there any way doctors can test for nerve damage?

A: There's a technique called **electromyography (EMG)**, which measures tiny electrical discharges from the muscles. It also conducts a nerve-conduction study, which measures the speed at which the nerves carry electrical signals.

The test is likely to be ordered if there is numbness, tingling or weakness in either of the arms or legs, suggesting that muscles and nerves are compromised. The muscle test also reveals whether muscles are degenerating or inflamed. If muscle weakness is limited to a particular location, it may be caused by the nerves that activate those muscles. For example, a disc may be pinching an adjacent nerve.

Q: What's actually done?

A: First, tiny needles are inserted into the muscles being assessed and the electrical currents are viewed on an oscilloscope screen. During the second part of the test, electrodes are placed on the skin for studying the nerves and a mild electric shock is sent down the nerve, revealing the speed at which nerve conduction takes place.

Q: Are there other tests?

A: There are a number of other procedures, testing everything from blood and urine to nerve conduction, that are used to evaluate a variety of back problems and screen out other disorders. They're described later in the book, along with those conditions. We'll conclude here by noting that a federal panel on acute low-back pain, convened by the U.S. Agency for Health Care Policy and Research, said last year that none of these tests should be ordered during the first three or four weeks of a problem unless a detailed physical examination and the patient's medical history indicate an underlying problem like nerve damage, tumors, fracture or dislocations.

2 MECHANICAL CAUSES OF BACK PAIN

Q: You've mentioned factors, like work and obesity, that can lead to back pain. But what's actually going on when my back hurts?

A: As we said in Chapter 1, it's often hard to state with any precision what is causing back pain. In fact, according to Augustus White, a prominent orthopedist at Harvard, up to 85 percent of back pain can't be definitively diagnosed. In his book, *Your Aching Back,* White notes, "In the strict scientific sense, modern medical science can definitely diagnose the cause in only about 15 percent of the acute cases."

This chapter is primarily about the most common—and, in many respects, the most difficult to diagnose—kinds of back pain: **strains, sprains, spasms** and disc problems. These are sometimes known as "mechanical" causes of back pain, because they relate to the mechanics of the back rather than to disease. We'll describe the conditions and how they can be treated conservatively—that is, without resorting to surgery.

There are a great many less common, and often more intractable, conditions associated with back pain.

We'll describe them in Chapter 3. In Chapter 4, we'll discuss surgical treatments for all back problems.

Q: Why is so little known about what causes and cures most back pain?

A: There are a number of reasons. The overwhelming obstacle to diagnosing back problems with any certainty is that there are often very weak correlations among the symptoms people report, the pathological findings and the imaging results, according to Richard A. Deyo, M.D., an internist at the University of Washington who is a leading researcher in back pain. People with severe back pain may have perfectly normal X-rays, for example, while disc problems show up on about 20 to 30 percent of imaging tests done on people without back pain.

And if you're not sure what you're treating, it's hard to know whether the treatment works. Most back-pain sufferers simply recover on their own. Psychosocial factors, which are believed to have a substantial influence on the onset of back pain, may also have a significant impact on recovery—but, because these are often overlooked in clinical trials and studies, it's hard to know how often the pain is mostly in one's head.

Finally, Deyo notes, it's difficult to select the appropriate outcomes in evaluating treatment. Almost no one ever dies from back pain and almost no one is "cured"; many people are left with occasional pains, somewhat circumscribed mobility and, in general, a back that's more vulnerable to another attack.

Q: Then if doctors don't know what's causing the problem, how can they treat it?

A: To some degree, the treatment of mechanical back problems particularly is a matter of trial and error, and—as we indicate in the discussion of treatment later in this chapter—what's tried has changed considerably over the years. In a recent article in the *New England Journal of Medicine,* Deyo put it even more harshly, stating that the history of medical care for low-back pain has been a series of fads in diagnosis and treatment.

Fortunately, as Harvard's White notes, "We doctors are actually better at managing your back problem than we are at finding its exact cause."

Q: Okay, no one knows exactly what's causing the pain. But what do they suspect?

A: That's another issue altogether. Most doctors will tell you that, in their experience, most back pain is due to an injury of muscle or ligament—which includes the annulus, or disc wall—or degenerative changes in the discs or facet joints. For example, Stephen Hochschuler, M.D., an orthopedic surgeon and cofounder of the Texas Back Institute, maintains in his book, *Back in Shape,* that 80 percent of all cases of back pain can be traced to one of three causes: muscle strain, **herniated discs** and facet joints.

Other doctors narrow the diagnosis even more. Robert L. Swezey, M.D., medical director of the Arthritis and Back Pain Center, in Santa Monica, California, goes so far as to say that about 95 percent of all low-back pain is a strain or sprain in the ligaments between the fourth and fifth lumbar vertebrae.

Such specificity would seem to be at odds with White's statement that medicine can diagnose only 15 percent of cases. But remember, he said "in the strict scientific sense."

STRAINS, SPRAINS AND SPASMS

Q: What's the difference between a strain and a sprain? And what about a spasm?

A: The term strain is used to describe an overworked or overstretched muscle, ligament, muscle or tendon, or one with a minor tear. Sprain refers to a more substantial tear. If you don't think that sounds like a significant difference, you may be reassured to note that doctors often have trouble distinguishing between them, too. However, the sudden sharp pain does let you know when your muscle is sprained or strained, not merely sore.

What's more distinctive is a spasm. You may have experienced the painful muscle contractions that people call a "charley horse." Well, muscles anywhere can go into spasm, but when it comes to your back it's usually the erector spinae muscles.

Q: Back to strains and sprains—what causes them?

A: When they come on suddenly, it's often from vigorous activity, such as sudden and unaccustomed exercise, or from an injury that occurs on the job or during sports, or from a fall or other accident.

However, strains and sprains don't have to come from exercise or a violent motion like a car crash. Sometimes if you twist or jerk your body the wrong way, you can tear a ligament or wrench an intervertebral facet joint, much like a knee joint. For that matter, you can develop a sprain from repeatedly assuming the same positions and making the same movements.

Q: Is it easy to strain or sprain a facet joint?

A: Fortunately, they're quite sturdy compared to, say, the joints in your fingers or toes. However, if the strain is severe enough, the joint may never recover fully, and may be strained more easily the next time it's subjected to stress.

Facet joint problems that result from aging, rather than from sprains or strains, are discussed in Chapter 3.

Q: What causes spasms?

A: A spasm is often a defensive reaction by the muscle to protect an injured area, so sprains, strains or any other back injury, including facet-joint and disc problems, often lead to spasms. Muscles also spasm around vertebrae when they fracture as the result of an accident or some of the diseases we describe in Chapter 3.

Q: You've been talking mainly about low-back problems. Don't strains, sprains or spasms ever develop in the neck?

A: They certainly do. One of the best-known conditions of this kind, when it involves the neck, is whiplash. Technically, that's a partial dislocation of the cervical vertebral facet joints, resulting in injury to the adjacent soft tissue. Sometimes the ligaments or muscles are strained or torn; less often the discs may be damaged.

Whiplash most often occurs when the head and neck are jerked violently. As you probably know, the usual cause is a head-on or, more likely, a rear-end car collision. As the head is thrown forward, the muscles in the back of the neck stretch rapidly, then contract violently, snapping the head backward. The damage occurs either through the rapid stretching or when the head snaps backward when the cervical muscles contract.

Q: What about psychological factors? Can stress cause back and neck strains and spasms?

A: Experts disagree. The official statement of the American Academy of Orthopaedic Surgeons (AAOS) is that emotional problems and stress-related tensions aren't a direct cause of low-back pain, but can certainly aggravate it. As the AAOS notes, "A person with low-back pain who is emotionally upset or stressed will often be very tense. Tension can increase spasms. These spasms lead to more pain, which itself causes the muscles to tighten or become tense."

However, many doctors believe that tension or stress is in fact the major cause of much back pain. Perhaps the leading exponent of that view is John Sarno, M.D., a physiatrist at New York University's Rusk Institute of Rehabilitation Medicine. Sarno believes that, more than 95 percent of the time, back pain comes from muscle spasms produced by tension.

So those are the two extremes. Somewhere in the middle is Augustus White, who predicts in *Your Aching Back* that "the future will most likely *prove* that stress . . . does indeed cause back pain."

Q: If tension does cause back spasms, how does it happen?

A: According to Sarno, tension—conscious or unconscious—causes constriction of the blood vessels that lead to the muscles and nerves in the back, and often to those in the shoulders and neck as well. The deprivation of blood, and of the oxygen it carries, can cause painful muscle spasms in both the low back and the neck. Sarno compares this to the situation of long-distance runners who suffer oxygen deprivation and develop leg cramps and spasm.

The pain itself creates fear, which prompts more tension and anxiety, and this leads to further constriction of the blood vessels. Sarno calls the condition tension myositis syndrome, or TMS.

Q: How are strains and sprains diagnosed—particularly if there's no sudden event, like a rear-end collision, to blame?

A: Unless someone has just been rear-ended or has just crawled off the dance floor, it's impossible to say with certainty that the problem is a sprain or strain. A CT scan may reveal a dislocated facet joint, but pulls and tears in soft tissue like muscles and ligaments don't show up on X-rays or other imaging technology the way bone or disc abnormalities do. However, a muscle that's gone into spasm may feel hard and swollen, like a knot.

So a strain or sprain is often a diagnosis by default—and hindsight, too: If the backache goes away spontaneously in a few days or weeks, the chances are good that it was caused by a sprain or strain.

DISC PROBLEMS

Q: What kinds of disc problems are there?

A: There's a variety of disc problems, but basically they're on a continuum—that is, they go from mild to severe as the condition or resiliency of the disc changes. As we mentioned in Chapter 1, discs are critical to the back's well-being because they separate the vertebrae and act as shock absorbers.

As a rule, disc problems begin with what's known as **disc degeneration** or degenerative disc disease. After the age of 30 or 40, discs gradually lose water, becoming less springy, smaller and less effective as shock absorbers. They may also become calcified; sometimes, but rarely, a bony fusion may grow across the disc. Typically this occurs at the junctures labeled L4-L5 and L5-S1—which, you'll recall from Chapter 1, means the low back.

Q: Is it painful?

A: Sometimes it is, sometimes it isn't. For reasons no one understands, people with identical X-rays —that is, discs that show the same extent of degeneration—may experience considerable back pain or no symptoms at all.

Q: You said there's a continuum. What happens as the degeneration gets worse?

A: The soft inside, or nucleus, of the disc pushes out beyond the normal confines of the retaining wall, and the disc begins to bulge against the ligament that holds it in place. When this happens, doctors say that the disc is herniating, or rupturing.

Whether or not this causes pain depends on how far the disc has bulged beyond its normal perimeter. Doctors measure the bulge in millimeters and talk about a 1-mm bulge or a 2-mm bulge. The larger the bulge, the more severe your symptoms.

Q: What's actually happening to the disc as it bulges?

A: There are a few stages of disc bulge:

- Early ruptures are known as **protrusions** or **prolapses**, when the disc bulges but no material escapes through the annulus.
- In an **extrusion**, the annulus tears and the nucleus breaks through into the spinal canal but remains connected.

• Finally, there's a condition known as **sequestration**, a complete herniation of the disc material through the annulus and the ligament. Nuclear material, known as **free fragments**, can move about in the spinal canal or the places where the nerves exit from the canal to the rest of the body.

Q: I suppose that's a slipped disc?

A: The phrase "slipped disc" is a misnomer: The discs themselves don't slip, because they're held in place by muscle and ligament even when part of the nucleus escapes.

Q: Who gets herniated discs?

A: Herniated discs are generally a stage in the progression of disc degeneration. According to the AAOS, most acute lumbar disc herniations occur in people between the ages of 35 and 55.

However, your discs don't have to be aging to herniate. They can also rupture as the result of trauma—car crashes, heavy lifting or other stress.

Q: How can I tell if I've got a herniated disc rather than, say, a muscle sprain?

A: Initially it may be hard to differentiate between the two—and sometimes you may have both. When the disc first begins to bulge, the back muscles may go into spasm to immobilize the area where the disc is pressing against the ligament.

Eventually, however, the bulging disc may be pushed against one of the nerves, or pinch it in some way. When that happens, you get a radiating pain called **radiculopathy** in whatever part of your body that's supplied by that nerve.

Q: Isn't the pain usually in the legs?

A: Yes, because the herniated disc is usually in the low back. It presses against the **sciatic nerve**, which runs from the lumbar spine through the leg to the foot. When that happens, people generally develop **sciatica**, a pain in the buttocks and down the back of the leg. It's such a sharp, searing pain that people tend to forget about any discomfort they felt in their back.

According to Richard Deyo, the likelihood of disc herniation in a patient without sciatica is one in 1,000.

Q: So herniated discs can be painful. But are they ever dangerous?

A: Certain massive disc herniations may cause compression of the spinal cord or cauda equina, the bundle of nerves that emerges from the spinal cord in the low back. Compression of the spinal cord, known as **cauda equina syndrome**, requires immediate surgery. Fortunately, the syndrome is quite rare, even in people with low-back pain.

There are a number of symptoms that tell you cauda equina syndrome is no ordinary back pain. The most consistent symptom is urinary retention, or difficulty urinating. Other warning signs include feelings of numbness and tingling sensations in the leg—possibly even a loss of sensation and function—and loss of bladder and bowel control.

Q: How do doctors or other practitioners diagnose herniated discs?

A: They start with a physical exam to check for nerve damage. That includes the straight-leg-raising test we mentioned in Chapter 1. They also look for **foot drop**, a condition in which people drag their feet because their leg muscles cannot raise their toes. Foot drop indicates that a ruptured disc is impinging on a nerve.

A doctor may also check for nerve damage by administering an electromyogram, described in Chapter 1. A slow conduction rate may indicate nerve damage from a protruding disc.

Q: Are there imaging techniques that show disc problems?

A: Yes. A couple are particularly useful. In a myelogram, the person lies on a table that's tilted while dye is injected into her spinal canal. The dye travels along the spine, filling the spaces surrounding the spinal nerves. On an X-ray, this shows whether herniated discs are impinging on the nerves. However, myelography has drawbacks: People who have it often find the procedure quite painful, and may also have excruciating headaches or backaches afterwards. There's also a risk of an acute allergic reaction to the dye used in one type of myelogram.

The other technique is a discogram, in which dye is injected directly into the disc. The dye would be trapped in a normal disc. If the disc has herniated, the dye leaks out into an adjoining area, shown on the X-ray. A discogram can be painful because it reproduces the pain created by the herniated disc.

Q: What about MRIs?

A: Magnetic resonance imaging (MRI) is widely used to diagnose disc problems, and to a degree it's replaced myelograms; it offers fewer complications and doesn't expose the individual to radiation. But between its cost and its ambiguous results, many experts believe even the MRI is used more than it should be.

One factor is that MRIs reveal ruptures that aren't causing any disability or discomfort. A research study led by Maureen C. Jensen, M.D., a radiologist at Hoag Memorial Hospital in Newport Beach, California, published in 1994 in the *New England Journal of Medicine,* found that, of 98 people *without* back pain, 52 percent had one or more bulging discs and 27 percent had protrusions, judging from their MRIs.

Without MRIs, these conditions would, and should, go untreated, experts say. But if someone's MRI reveals a ruptured disc and the person has back pain, many doctors automatically assume a cause-and-effect and give the wrong treatment.

Q: You've been talking mostly about lumbar discs. Don't discs in the cervical or thoracic spine herniate?

A: Yes, although herniated discs are far less common in the neck than in the low back, and rarer still in the midback. In fact, thoracic disc herniations are so rare that their symptoms—a tightening of the chest and severe radiating pain around the rib cage—are often mistakenly attributed to non-spine-related problems.

Cervical discs herniate about one-third as often as low-back discs and, like thoracic disc problems, may be harder to diagnose. Possibly because the neck is constantly moving, **osteophytes** often form in this area. When there's nerve pain, it's not always clear whether it's a disc or an osteophyte that's pressing on the nerve.

Q: What causes cervical disc problems?

A: In addition to accidents, the telephone is a common culprit, particularly among computer users. People hold the phone with an upraised shoulder while they type—or, for that matter, while they cook, write or do anything else that requires both hands.

Twisting one's neck this way can damage the C5/C6 or C6/C7 discs in the neck, leading to cervical radiculopathy—a condition that Emil Pascarelli, M.D., director of ambulatory care at St. Luke's-Roosevelt Hospital in New York City, calls "phone shoulder syndrome." In addition to neck pain, it can cause weakness in the shoulder and upper arm, and possibly numbness in the fingers.

TREATMENT

Q: How are all these conditions treated?

A: In the vast majority of cases, conservative—that is, nonsurgical—treatment provides significant relief, in terms of both reducing pain and improving mobility. However, there's a great range of conservative measures: physical measures (bed rest, exercise, spinal manipulation and braces), oral medication, injectable drugs and counter-stimulation such as heat and cold, **transcutaneous electrical nerve stimulation (TENS)** and acupuncture.

As you can see, it's a list of many options, and there's a changing consensus in the medical community about the value of the items on it. For example, in its recent report, the Agency for Health Care Policy and Research panel on low-back pain put an official stamp of approval on the "less-is-more" approach; it endorsed aspirin, exercise and spinal manipulation over prescription drugs and bed rest. The panel said that, of the estimated $20 billion spent in direct medical costs for low back problems in 1990, about $7 billion might have been spent needlessly on services that did little good.

In this chapter, we'll describe state-of-the-art approaches to back pain by experts in the field. You may find that some of these are in conflict with the more traditional practices of your family doctor or other providers whom you consult. You can question both the old wisdom and the new: In back pain, as we've indicated earlier, not much is certain.

For a copy of the agency's booklet, "Understanding Acute Low Back Problems," call (800) 358-9295 or write P.O. Box 8547, Silver Spring, MD 20907.

Q: Do I really need to see a doctor or other back-care specialist?

A: As we noted in Chapter 1, the vast majority of people who get back pain recover on their own, without consulting anyone. Unless you have certain symptoms—typically, pain radiating down an arm or leg, indicating a pinched nerve—you can try treating the problem yourself with the measures described below. Most simple back pain will improve within a day or two; if it doesn't, seek professional help.

Bed Rest

Q: Okay, if my back starts hurting, what's the first thing I should do?

A: ''Stop what you're doing,'' says Hochschuler of the Texas Back Institute. In his book, *Back in Shape,* Hochschuler notes, ''Many people persist in whatever they're doing even after they get a sudden burst of back pain. In fact, they should immediately stop what they're doing and rest.''

Q: Just fall into bed?

A: Your back will recover best when you lie on your back or side, with hips and knees bent; for certain conditions you may even lie on your back with your legs raised and bent at the knee over a chair. Sleeping on your stomach, because it puts your back in a hyperextension position, isn't a great idea; if you must do it, experts say, put a pillow under your pelvic bone to straighten your spine.

Q: How much bed rest is advisable?

A: The new medical wisdom is that only two or three days should suffice for the vast majority of people whose acute back pain is due to the garden variety of sprains, strains or spasms. If your back-care provider believes your pain is due to compressed nerves, usually from a herniated disc, she may recommend more bed rest—perhaps 7 to 10 days.

In the past, patients with low-back pain were told to go to bed until their pain subsided. As a result, their muscles lost conditioning and began to atrophy, or waste away. Treatment now encourages patients to start moving as soon as possible. In fact, a recent study in Finland, published in the *New England Journal of Medicine,* found that acute-low-back patients who continued ordinary activities—as much as their pain permitted—recovered faster than people who had brief bed rest.

Exercise

Q: But wouldn't that just aggravate the condition?

A: No. In fact, exercise is now generally regarded as one of the best and fastest ways to relieve back pain and restore mobility.

For one thing, it's believed that exercise stimulates the production of endorphins, the body's natural painkillers. When people don't exercise, their endorphin levels fall.

Secondly, exercise that is moderately aerobic improves the flow of blood and oxygen to discs, joints and muscles, accelerating the healing process. Hochschuler notes that breaking into a little sweat indicates you're raising the temperature of the muscle tissues, relaxing painful spasms.

Q: What kind of exercise should I do?

A: Before starting an exercise program, consult the physician, chiropractor or other health-care provider who's treating your back. She'll probably recommend low-impact aerobic exercises. Walking, bicycling (mobile or stationary) and/or swimming (with the possible exception of the butterfly stroke, which forces you to arch your back) are all good for you and your back. In fact, any exercise in water—which provides support as well as resistance to movement—can be good for you.

Alternatively, you may prefer to start with "floor" exercises, of which there are two main categories: **extension** and **flexion**—just like the two main kinds of muscles described in Chapter 1.

Q: What are some extension exercises?

A: In *Back in Shape,* Hochschuler describes the basic extension exercise, the press-up, as follows: "For the person in acute back pain, start by lying face down or [on your stomach, resting] on your elbows for 3 to 5 minutes. At first, your arms may have to be bent as you press up. Try to work up to where you can straighten your arms completely. The first few press-ups may be uncomfortable, but pain should lessen with subsequent sessions."

Q: What are some flexion exercises?

A: There's a greater variety of those. Here are two of the most common, as described by Hochschuler:

- "Pelvic tilt. Lie on back with knees raised and arms extended [outward]. Press the low back down against the floor by tightening the abdominal muscles, squeezing the buttocks and rolling top of pelvis backward. Hold for 10 seconds.

- "Single knee to chest. Lie on back and lift one knee to the chest. Repeat with other leg. Hold for 10 seconds. Remember to keep your low back in contact with the floor."

Q: Aren't there any exercises that combine flexion and extension?

A: There's one widely used exercise you probably already know; perhaps you've heard it described as "the cat" or "the angry cat." Get on all fours on the floor and pull in your abdominal muscles. First, drop your head forward and round your back as you tilt your pelvis. Then raise your head and slowly arch your back.

Q: Are these exercises good for the various back problems, from sprains to herniated discs?

A: In theory, all of these exercises are good for bulging—but not completely herniated—discs because they help recentralize the soft nucleus. By extending backward, the vertebrae may gently push the nucleus back into position and relieve the stress on nearby nerves. Flexion exercises help restore flexibility.

In fact, muscle-strain injuries and disc problems tend to respond better to extension exercises. In some cases, flexion exercises may increase pain. On the other hand, people with facet-joint problems often feel much better when they do flexion exercises and worse when they do extension exercises.

In Chapter 3, we'll describe the appropriate exercises for other conditions.

Q: But what if these exercises hurt?

A: If they hurt *a lot,* don't do them. In *Back in Shape,* Hochschuler offers two guidelines for his basic exercise regimen:

1. "If your back begins to hurt worse with a specific exercise, stop doing it.

2. "If you can't straighten up fully or perform any of these first-aid exercises without severe pain, stick to bed rest. And if your pain is this disabling, it may be a signal to visit a back specialist to rule out any serious back injury."

Of course, pain is highly subjective. Most people who exercise after a back injury experience what doctors would term only "discomfort," especially if their backs are extremely sore and if they weren't used to exercising before they got injured. In that case, they'll have to endure the discomfort before they can benefit from the exercise.

Q: Are there any other exercises that are good for the back?

A: Yoga, which may be loosely described as an exercise (as well as a relaxation technique), isn't generally cited by doctors as an exercise for back pain but some people swear by it. In a survey more than a decade ago of some 500 chronic-back-pain sufferers, by market researcher (and back-pain sufferer) Arthur C. Klein and science writer Dava Sobel, the practitioner category that scored highest was yoga instructor (with a 96 percent rating for "moderate to dramatic" long-term relief).

Spinal Manipulation

Q: You said earlier that spinal manipulation is more widely accepted than it was. Are there any studies that say whether it's effective?

A: Yes, and these studies have given it unexpectedly high marks. (Just to remind you, spinal manipulation is the practice—primarily by chiropractors but also by osteopaths and even some orthopedists—of applying pressure to the spine to restore alignment and mobility.)

In 1991, Rand, the research organization based in Santa Monica, California, conducted a study that concluded that manipulation was indeed an appropriate therapy for patients with certain types of low-back pain. It said the best candidates were people whose pain had lasted less than three weeks, who had no signs of spinal nerve damage and whose spines appeared to be normal in X-rays.

In studies reviewed by Rand, people in this group had significant relief after manipulation and were able to return to work sooner than similar patients treated with more conventional treatment such as bed rest or painkillers.

However, the expert panel, which included medical doctors, osteopaths and chiropractors, was divided on the value of manipulation for chronic—as opposed to acute—low-back pain.

Q: Did the study recommend how long manipulation should be tried?

A: According to Paul Shekelle, M.D., the Rand researcher and internist who led the study, the research indicated that three to six weeks of manipulation provided short-term relief for acute back pain. In general, the panel agreed that, if manipulation didn't produce an improvement within four weeks or so, it should be abandoned in favor of other treatments.

Q: Are there any other studies that support—or don't support—the value of manipulation?

A: The federal panel on low-back pain, which reviewed more than 3,900 studies, also found spinal manipulation helpful, especially during the first four weeks of pain. Like the Rand study, the federal task force study looked at manipulation generally, not chiropractic spinal adjustment.

People who have been treated by manipulation seem to give it mixed reviews. For example, in a 1989 survey of members of Group Health of Puget Sound, a health maintenance organization, chiropractors received substantially more favorable reviews: 66 percent of chiropractors' patients were "very satisfied" with their care, compared with 22 percent of physicians' patients.

However, the researchers cautioned that chiropractors' high ratings might reflect their bedside manner as much as the quality of care they deliver. Chiropractors were thought to be more concerned about their patients, believed the pain was real and were confident about the diagnosis and treatment.

And in the Klein/Sobel survey we cited earlier, 28 percent of those who answered the questionnaire said chiropractors provided "moderate to dramatic" long-term relief, while another 28 percent said chiropractors provided temporary relief only; 33 percent said they'd gotten no relief, and 11 percent said they felt worse afterward. (Admittedly, those rankings still put them ahead of orthopedists, neurosurgeons and family practitioners in the survey.)

Braces and Traction

Q: When people get whiplash, they're in a neck brace for weeks. Do braces really work?

A: There's no hard evidence that lumbar braces are effective in treating back pain, according to the federal panel. The anecdotal evidence is mixed.

Many people, health-care providers as well as patients, fear that the brace will be used as a crutch—that the patient will become dependent on it and not perform exercises to rehabilitate her back. But others believe a back or neck brace can help the body heal and facilitate rehabilitation. "By using bracing, I have avoided surgery in a high percentage of my patients," says Lyle Micheli, M.D., an orthopedic surgeon at Harvard Medical School.

In Chapter 5, we'll discuss some specific kinds of braces and other back and neck supports that may be used for preventing or easing back pain.

Q: What about traction?

A: Traction, which is a force applied along the axis of the spine in an attempt to elongate it, sometimes provides temporary relief from pain caused by a disc pressing on a nerve. But it doesn't push a herniated disc back into place, and it's been largely discredited as a cure for back problems.

That's also true of so-called gravity boots, a form of gravity traction in which the spine is elongated by hanging the hapless individual upside down. In fact, gravity boots have been known to cause damage, including bleeding in the back of the eye and sudden increases in blood pressure.

Medication

Q: What medications are commonly used to treat back pain?

A: At one time, prescription medication such as muscle relaxants, narcotic analgesics and sleeping pills were standard fare for acute back pain. While that remains the practice of a great many physicians, the new thinking of the medical community—epitomized in the report of the federal panel on low-back pain—is that, as with bed rest, "the less, the better."

"My approach in 1981 was to always give medicine," says Thomas B. Curtis, a physical medicine and rehabilitation specialist at Virginia Mason Medical Center, in Seattle, Washington. "Now I usually don't give any."

When physicians do prescribe, they're more careful to limit the dosage to a few days because of concern about physical dependence and other risks.

Q: So what do these doctors say I should take to kill the pain?

A: The federal panel recommended a handful of oral over-the-counter medications that, it said, were usually adequate to control pain while keeping the back-pain sufferer as active as possible. Specifically, it mentioned acetaminophen (Tylenol or Datril) and **nonsteroidal anti-inflammatory drugs (NSAIDs)**, including aspirin and **ibuprofen** (Advil, Nuprin, Medipren, Motrin IB and Ibuprin).

Q: How do they compare?

A: In terms of reducing muscle swelling or **inflammation**, ibuprofen is the most effective, followed by aspirin; acetaminophen trails in third place. However, aspirin is more effective than ibuprofen as a painkiller, according to Hochschuler and other physicians.

Q: What about side effects?

A: They all have drawbacks. The most frequent complication of aspirin and ibuprofen is gastrointestinal (GI) irritation. Aspirin also can interfere with blood coagulating and result in abnormal bleeding in some circumstances.

To avoid GI problems, you can take certain brands, like Ecotrin, that are coated, or take the medicine rectally. Although doctors often advise you to take these medications with meals, it's not clear that it helps. In addition, a prescription drug called misoprostol (Cytotec, made by G.D. Searle) has been shown to block most of the gastrointestinal problems caused by NSAIDs.

Q: If aspirin and ibuprofen have all those side effects, should I take acetaminophen instead?

A: Only in moderation. A recent study published in the *New England Journal of Medicine* found that taking just one Tylenol or other acetaminophen daily for at least a year may double the risk of kidney failure. Admittedly, the researchers, from the Johns Hopkins School of Public Health, noted that kidney damage is rare even among heavy users; they estimated that heavy use of acetaminophen to relieve pain may cause about 5,000 cases of kidney failure in the United States each year.

A second study, published in the *Journal of the American Medical Association,* reported that, when it's taken after a fast or by people who are heavy drinkers, acetaminophen in even moderate amounts can damage the liver.

Q: What if these over-the-counter drugs don't help? Don't doctors prescribe anything?

A: A number of stronger NSAIDs are available by prescription only, such as nabumetone (Relafen, made by SmithKline Beecham).

Like aspirin and ibuprofen, these drugs tend to cause GI problems. A couple have been associated with particularly serious side effects: phenylbutazone, which has been associated with bone-marrow suppression; and indomethacin (Indocin, from Merck), which has a higher reported incidence of gastrointestinal side effects. Otherwise, according to the federal panel on low back problems, there's no significant demonstrated difference among the NSAIDs in terms of prevalence or severity of complications.

Q: My doctor always prescribes muscle relaxants when my back goes into spasm. What's wrong with that?

A: While they're still widely prescribed, the new thinking by experts such as the federal panel on low-back problems is that they're no more effective than NSAIDs, and they have other side effects—about one-third of the people who take them become drowsy. Augustus White argues that spasms generally subside on their own once the pain and inflammation have subsided. And the relaxants haven't even been proven specifically to relax muscles.

However, if your spasms persist, your doctor might prescribe a muscle relaxant such as cyclobenzaprine (Flexeril, made by Merck) or methocarbamol (Robaxin, made by A.H. Robins) and tranquilizers such as diazepam (Valium and Librium, from Roche).

Q: Aren't there any other drugs that are more effective than aspirin?

A: When the pain is particularly severe, some doctors prescribe painkillers such as acetaminophen with codeine. However, as the federal panel warned, the side effects can be significant: dizziness and nausea, fatigue, impaired vision and difficulty concentrating, as well as the potential for physical dependence.

Many back-pain experts also try short courses of high-dose oral steroids, or **corticosteroids**, such as cortisone and prednisone, to reduce pain and inflammation. These have side effects, too, including increased appetite and weight gain, sudden mood swings, restlessness and nervousness, trouble sleeping, increased body hair, and a lowered resistance to bacterial and yeast infections. While the federal panel said that some of these effects can be reduced or eliminated by taking the steroids every other day, it advised against the use of such steroids for acute low-back problems.

Q: Are these drugs ever injected?

A: Injections of cortisone into discs and facet joints, to reduce inflammation, have been popular for a number of years, but their efficacy has never been established. A study published in the Oct. 3, 1991, *New England Journal of Medicine* found that corticosteroid injections into facet joints were barely more effective than placebos in treating chronic low-back pain.

Harvard's White advises against such injections, arguing that cortisone may irritate structures and may even accelerate arthritis. However, John Frymoyer, a leading orthopedic researcher, has suggested that the injections may have some value in providing a brief respite from motion-limiting pain to allow the individual to start exercising.

Q: Aren't there other drugs that are injected into back muscles?

A: You may be thinking of so-called trigger-point injections, which involve the injection of local anesthetic and/or other substances—glycerin, dextrose and water are often combined—into muscles and ligaments near tender areas along the spine. The theory is that this stimulates the formation of scar tissue and blood flow, helping the soft tissue to repair.

While such injections are widely used, they were not recommended by the federal panel on acute low-back pain. The panel said their efficacy appears "equivocal" and that they can have serious complications, including damage to nerves or other tissues, infection and hemorrhage.

Q: What about antidepressants? Are they ever prescribed?

A: Physicians do prescribe antidepressant medications to people with low-back pain in the belief that the medications will reduce pain, help them get the sleep they need, and alleviate the depression that often occurs with chronic pain. Amitriptyline (Elavil, made by Roche) is sometimes prescribed to reduce radicular pain.

How effective they are, however, isn't clear. Again, the federal panel was doubtful, noting that studies of people with chronic low-back problems found that antidepressants weren't significantly more effective than placebos.

Counter-Stimulation

Q: You mentioned heat and cold as "counter-stimulation" treatment. What do you mean?

A: It's believed that certain treatments work on the nervous system to block—temporarily—the pain signals from your back. Acupuncture, TENS, heat and cold, and massage are all believed to "counter-stimulate" or "counter-irritate" the nervous system, modifying pain perception.

Q: Okay, then should I use a heating pad?

A: Actually, the new rule of thumb is ice, then heat. Experts recommend applying ice to the painful area for 20 minutes every two hours, in the first 48 hours after the pain flares up, to reduce swelling, slow inflammation and relieve soreness. Cold also acts as an anesthetic by numbing sore tissues. (To avoid a skin "burn," use an ice pack.)

Essentially, the cold contracts the veins, reducing circulation. Once you stop applying cold, the veins overcompensate and dilate, allowing blood to rush into the sore area. This blood, along with the oxygen it carries, begins healing the damaged tissue.

Follow with heat—dry or moist—to promote healing by increasing circulation and relaxing muscle spasms.

Q: Do liniments help?

A: Liniments, like heat and cold, are "counter-stimulants" that work indirectly to relieve pain. The heat that a liniment like Ben-Gay (made by Pfizer) produces doesn't actually reach the muscle. Instead it causes a burning sensation on the skin, helping block the pain signals from the sprain or strain.

Q: What about massage?

A: Like heat and cold, massage may somehow block pain transmission or it may cause local circulatory changes under the skin. Massage therapists work on the soft tissue of the back rather than on the spine itself, kneading muscle to reduce stiffness and pain. Because massage increases circulation, it can help accelerate the repair of damaged tissue.

Q: How does acupuncture block pain?

A: Acupuncturists, following techniques developed in China thousands of years ago, use thin needles—sometimes accompanied by low-voltage electric current—to locate and treat pain, presumably by affecting the central nervous system.

Q: Is it effective?

A: While there's plenty of support for acupuncture, it's purely anecdotal. The federal panel on low-back problems couldn't find any research establishing its effectiveness. But in the Klein/Sobel survey we cited earlier, acupuncturists do significantly better than chiropractors, orthopedists and neurologists—although well below yoga instructors—in their ability to treat back pain.

Q: You mentioned some kind of electrical stimulation called TENS. What's that?

A: TENS (transcutaneous electrical nerve stimulation) is a widely used treatment for chronic back pain that involves administering pulses of low-voltage electric current, through electrodes taped to the body. The theory is that, like acupuncture, it works by stimulating the body's endorphins, or internal pain-control substances.

Q: Does it work?

A: No more than a placebo, according to a recent study by Richard Deyo and other researchers. The study, which was published in the June 7, 1990, *New England Journal of Medicine,* compared the effectiveness of TENS with a program of stretching exercises for people with chronic low-back pain. It found that after one month TENS had no clinically significant effect, while exercise had helped substantially. In a follow-up two months after treatment stopped, only those people who continued to exercise maintained the improvement they'd made earlier.

Q: So, when all's said and done, exercise is the best treatment?

A: There's no statistical proof that exercise is the single best therapy. For example, a study of almost 300 back- and neck-pain sufferers, reported in the *British Medical Journal* in 1992, found that non-traditional techniques in general—exercise, massage, heat and spinal manipulation—provided the most relief from pain symptoms. But increasingly, clinicians, based on experience, are recommending exercise as the primary treatment.

Chemonucleolysis

Q: Are there any treatments specifically for ruptured discs?

A: There's a rather controversial procedure known as **chemonucleolysis**, in which an enzyme called **chymopapain** is injected into the nucleus of a bulging disc. Chymopapain, an enzyme found in the papaya plant, is the same substance used in meat tenderizers, and it has the same effect: It breaks down protein.

While chemonucleolysis isn't a surgical procedure, it's typically performed by a surgeon in a hospital, using a long needle, guided by an X-ray machine and with the patient under a general anesthetic.

Q: Why is it controversial?

A: There's a one in 100 chance that chymopapain will trigger a potentially fatal allergic reaction known as anaphylactic shock, in which the blood pressure drops rapidly. While that sounds alarming, doctors can reduce the likelihood of this reaction by testing patients for allergic sensitivity before the procedure. And hospitals should be prepared to deal with a reaction promptly, before it becomes serious.

There are other important limits on the use of chymopapain. It cannot be used when the disc has herniated completely and disc fragments are floating in the spinal canal. And, because of its potentially toxic nature, it cannot be given twice to the same individual in a lifetime. Furthermore, because the procedure can produce severe back spasms, recovery can be painful for weeks.

Q: Is it an effective treatment?

A: It's reportedly successful approximately 75 percent of the time. But the relief may be relatively brief: By dissolving the nucleus, which is the intended result, chemonucleolysis can accelerate the aging process of the disc and trigger other problems down the road.

Because of such drawbacks, many people—clinicians and back-pain sufferers—may prefer surgery to treat disc problems that conservative therapy can't help. Chapter 4 describes surgical approaches to herniated discs.

3 OTHER TYPES OF BACK PAIN

Q: Okay, that takes care of the most common kinds of back pain—muscle, joint and disc problems. What's left?

A: A lot. There are a great many other conditions that cause back pain and, while they're not as common as sprains or spasms, you've probably heard of most of them and even known people who have them. They include arthritis, **osteoporosis**, spinal curvatures such as **scoliosis**, and systemic diseases such as cancer and infection. In addition, there are disorders that occur elsewhere in the body but produce what's known as "referred pain" in the back.

In this chapter, we'll describe all these conditions and how they can be treated conservatively. In Chapter 4 we'll discuss surgical treatments for these conditions as well as for disc problems.

ARTHRITIS

Q: How does arthritis affect backs?

A: Arthritis is inflammation of a joint, or several joints, and inflammation almost always brings pain. When arthritis occurs in the back, it can take a variety of forms.

The most common of these is **osteoarthritis**, also called **spondylitis** (Greek for "inflammation of the vertebra") or **degenerative arthritis**. Often found in elderly people, it's known more colloquially as a "wear-and-tear" arthritis.

Another fairly common, but far more crippling condition is **rheumatoid arthritis**. And there are some relatively rare arthritic conditions, such as **ankylosing spondylitis**, that we'll also discuss in this chapter.

Osteoarthritis

Q: Let's start with osteoarthritis. What's that like?

A: Osteoarthritis typically involves inflammation of the facet joints between vertebrae. Over time —and particularly if you've had an injury—the cartilage in joints degenerates, causing pain and inflammation. Sometimes the synovial tissue that lines and lubricates the joints also becomes irritated or inflamed. The muscles may also go into spasm, which increases the pain.

Most people's joints succumb to wear and tear over the years, but not everybody has pain. According to the National Institute of Arthritis, Musculoskeletal and Skin Disorders, which is part of the National Institutes of Health, almost everyone over the age of 60 has some form of osteoarthritis, but only about half feel pain and stiffness.

For a smaller, not as lucky fraction of individuals, osteoarthritis may result in a condition called **spinal stenosis**, which we'll discuss shortly.

Q: How can I tell whether I've got osteoarthritis?

A: There are a number of symptoms that suggest osteoarthritis:

- Your pain is worse when you've been inactive for a time, such as when you get up in the morning.
- Your back aches more when the weather is cold or damp or the barometric pressure changes.
- You're increasingly stiff or inflexible, regardless of the time of day.
- Your spine hurts from bending, lifting, prolonged sitting, twisting or riding in vibrating vehicles.

X-rays can substantiate the symptoms. The likely diagnosis is osteoarthritis if there's no other explanation for your back pain and your X-rays reveal minor deformities of the vertebrae as well as the formation of osteophytes, or spurs, around the edges of the vertebrae.

Q: How is it treated?

A: While you can't prevent osteoarthritis, if you're in good shape you can usually keep it from becoming painful. That means exercising in moderation but regularly, maintaining good muscle tone and controlling your weight; at this stage, you may opt for treatment by a chiropractor rather than a physician. If the condition does become painful, you can take one of the anti-inflammatory drugs discussed in Chapter 2. Occasionally doctors recommend wearing a brace.

For some people, osteoarthritis is confined to one area of the back and causes persistent pain and immobility. In that case, your doctor may try a short series of injections of small amounts of cortisonelike drugs to reduce pain and inflammation. If they don't help, surgery may be an option.

Spinal Stenosis

Q: You said osteoarthritis can cause spinal stenosis. What is that?

A: Spinal stenosis is a degenerative condition in which the spinal column gradually encroaches upon the spinal canal, pressing on the nerves that run through it. Pain radiates along the path of these compressed nerves. As a result, the pain of stenosis is more acute where the nerve leads to—typically, the legs—than in the back itself.

Stenosis can affect any part of the spine, but it's usually concentrated in the low back. (That's why you may hear the term "lumbar stenosis" instead of spinal stenosis.) The typical person with spinal stenosis is a man in his 50s or 60s.

Q: How can I tell if I have spinal stenosis?

A: People who get spinal stenosis often have hints, like bouts of back or leg pain, years before the condition becomes serious. Other early symptoms are more nebulous. Your legs might feel a bit odd, weak or rubbery, or like they might "give out" on you when you're walking.

The classic symptom of stenosis is leg pain, usually in both legs at the same time. It may be brought on by walking or even by standing still. Straightening the spine compresses the nerves and exacerbates the pain, while bending over or sitting eases it. That's why people with spinal stenosis often tend to walk bent forward. It hurts more to walk downhill or down a flight of stairs, because you have to lean back slightly, than to walk uphill or upstairs, when you lean forward.

As the condition worsens, even sitting can become painful. The pain may wake you up at night. Eventually it can become so severe that it's immobilizing.

Q: How is it diagnosed?

A: Through the usual assortment of physical and imaging tests. The straight-leg-raising test is one important diagnostic tool, because it separates people with lumbar disc problems (who can't raise their legs) from people with spinal stenosis (who can). X-rays may show some disc collapse or arthritic changes in the spine, but a CT scan or MRI is necessary to determine just where and how much the canal has been narrowed.

Q: Is osteoarthritis the only cause of spinal stenosis?

A: No, but it's the most common. Some people may be more predisposed to spinal stenosis because they were born with a comparatively narrow canal. Furthermore, anything that encroaches on the spinal canal can lead to stenosis, and that includes herniated discs. The most famous case of spinal stenosis is probably that of Joe Montana, the professional quarterback whose stenosis was aggravated by injured discs which were ultimately treated surgically.

Certain other diseases, such as **Paget's disease of the bone** (a disorder, often associated with osteoarthritis, in which the bones may weaken and fracture easily) and **fluoridosis** (due to excessive fluoride, which can thicken bone), may also cause or contribute to stenosis. And stenosis can sometimes be an unfortunate complication of spinal surgery.

Q: Is surgery like Montana's the preferred treatment for spinal stenosis?

A: No, it's a last resort. ''Montana's case was one in 100,'' says the man who performed the surgery, Arthur White, M.D., medical director of the San Francisco Spine Institute at Seton Medical Center in Daly

City, California. The reason White chose to operate, he explains, is that other treatments had failed and Montana was in so much pain he couldn't walk.

In general, White and other physicians recommend a more conservative approach: bed rest (preferably on your side or back, with hips and knees bent), pain-killers, anti-inflammatory drugs, a corset or brace that holds your spine in a flexed position and decreases spinal movement, and gradual exercise like the bent-knee sit-up, which strengthens your abdominal muscles. Chiropractors maintain that many cases of spinal stenosis also respond to chiropractic. If conservative measures don't produce a gradual improvement, however, then surgery may be inevitable.

Rheumatoid Arthritis

Q: On to rheumatoid arthritis. What's that all about?

A: Rheumatoid arthritis (RA) is a chronic condition in which the immune system essentially turns on itself, so that the body behaves as though it were fighting a foreign substance. When it affects the back, the joints in the lumbar spine or the neck may become inflamed and eventually damaged. The disease can also spread to the connective tissue almost anywhere in the body.

Q: Is it common?

A: About 2 percent of the population have rheumatoid arthritis, and only 10 percent of those people have severe joint problems. In other words, only two people out of a thousand have severe joint problems from rheumatoid arthritis. And in most cases, it occurs in the knee, hip, hand and wrist joints, less often in the back.

It affects women two or three times more often than men, and typically in middle age.

Q: How is it diagnosed?

A: In its initial stages, rheumatoid arthritis can be difficult to diagnose. The symptoms may be very mild, and doctors may confuse RA with several other diseases that produce inflammation.

When the disease is well established, it's easy to diagnose through joint deformity that shows up on X-rays. There are also a few blood tests doctors may perform: a complete blood count (partly to screen out other conditions), an **erythrocyte sedimentation rate** test—or "sed rate" test—and a test for rheumatoid factor.

The sed rate test, by measuring how quickly red blood cells cling together and settle to the bottom of a test tube, indicates the degree of inflammation. The rheumatoid factor test also signals the presence of inflammation. However, neither is a definitive test for RA.

Q: How is rheumatoid arthritis treated?

A: There's no cure for RA, merely ways to control its progression and pain. Aspirin, other NSAIDs and steroids can help limit the inflammation and pain. Other treatments mentioned in Chapter 2, including braces, gentle exercise and heat and cold, may prevent progressive deformity. Some people with RA also receive **gold salts**—injections or oral doses of gold compounds. Chiropractic is inappropriate for RA.

Researchers in England are studying two new drugs that have shown promising short-term results against RA by blocking a protein said to trigger swelling. However, they're both in the developmental stage.

Ankylosing Spondylitis

Q: You mentioned another arthritic condition, ankylosing spondylitis. What's that?

A: It's a painful and potentially crippling form of arthritis in which a bony bridge forms between the vertebrae—thus "ankylosing," or fusing, portions of the spine.

The first symptoms are a stiffness in the low back and sacroiliac, particularly in the morning, which eases with any movement. The condition may progress rapidly up the spine in some people, not at all in others.

Sometimes the disease will fuse just a few of the lower lumbar vertebrae; in others all the vertebrae may become fused. The connection between the ribs and the thoracic spine may become so rigid that the person with ankylosing spondylitis can barely expand his chest. Some people may be forced to walk or sit in a slightly crouched position; others are so bent over they face the ground and can't turn their heads from side to side.

Q: Who gets it?

A: Ankylosing spondylitis is a young man's disease; it typically surfaces in men in their 20s and 30s, although it may afflict them for decades. Preliminary research indicates there's a genetic factor.

Q: How is it diagnosed?

A: It's hard to diagnose when it begins. A doctor would probably start with a physical examination and a sed rate test. However, some people with this condition still have normal sed rates. And there are several other arthritic conditions, including **Reiter's syndrome**, that also produce a high sedimentation rate.

There is a somewhat more precise test called HLA-B27, which tests for the presence of a specific protein, called B-27, on the surface of their white blood cells. Ninety percent of white people with ankylosing spondylitis test positive. But not even this test is foolproof: 10 percent of white people and a higher percent of nonwhites with this condition will test negative—and even more people will have false-positive results.

Q: What about X-rays?

A: Ankylosing spondylitis does show up on X-rays in various ways: changes in the sacroiliac joints and ossified discs that bulge slightly—creating a pattern that doctors call "bamboo spine." However, these aren't always apparent in the early stages of the disease.

Q: How is it treated?

A: There's no known way to prevent or cure ankylosing spondylitis, but it is important to start treating it as soon as it's diagnosed, to try to slow the disease's progression. People are told to watch their posture, practice deep breathing, and do special exercises to keep their spines supple. Sometimes they wear braces to prevent major deformity.

In its acute or inflamed stages, ankylosing spondylitis should be treated by a physician. If severe deformity occurs, surgery may be recommended.

Q: I've read about some man who cured himself of this condition. How did he do it?

A: You're probably referring to Norman Cousins, the late *Saturday Review* editor who claimed to cure himself of ankylosing spondylitis with "laughter therapy." In his book *Anatomy of an Illness As Perceived by the Patient,* he describes how he treated his condition successfully by checking into a hotel room and watching hour after hour of old "Candid Camera" programs and Marx Brothers movies. He also took megadoses of vitamin C.

How did it work? In his book *Your Aching Back,* orthopedic surgeon Augustus White suggests that Cousins may have felt better because he stimulated his brain to produce endorphins.

OSTEOPOROSIS

Q: What's osteoporosis? Isn't that what old women get?

A: Yes, though you're not immune if you're an elderly male. Osteoporosis, which literally means "porous bones," is a disease of progressive bone loss associated with an increased risk of fractures. It's a major health problem, affecting 25 million Americans and contributing to an estimated 1.3 million bone fractures per year. One in two women and one in five men over the age of 65 will eventually sustain bone fractures due to osteoporosis.

Obviously, those aren't all in the back—fractures of the hip, wrist, arm and leg as well as the spine are all too common when elderly people take a tumble or even engage in a task like opening a window that's stuck.

The risk of these "compression fractures," as they're called, increases with age. According to Stephen Hochschuler of the Texas Back Institute, it's been estimated that half of all women over the age of 80 have evidence of vertebral fractures. Osteoporosis is usually to blame, although compression fractures sometimes occur in people with cancer that involves the bone.

Q: Does the back pain come from the fractures?

A: In part. Experts believe that, when a vertebra fractures, the surrounding muscles go into spasm. Once the fracture heals, usually through conservative care such as bed rest and painkillers, the pain subsides. However, people with osteoporosis may also be in pain or incapacitated because the disease shrinks and curves their spine, squeezing their lungs and making it difficult to breathe.

Q: What causes osteoporosis?

A: No one really knows, though they do know that the aging process is a critical component. Everyone loses bone with age and, after 35, the body builds less new bone to replace losses of old bone. Bones become thinner—less ''dense,'' in medical parlance—and more fragile.

Q: But don't more women than men have osteoporosis?

A: Yes. Women begin to lose bone rapidly—up to 2 percent annually—with the onset of menopause and the decline in their levels of estrogens, or female hormones.

Furthermore, women don't have to be older to develop this condition. Women who undergo early menopause or amenorrhea (the absence of menstruation) are also candidates for osteoporosis. Amenorrhea can be caused by excessive exercise—running much more than 20 miles a week, for example—as well as by eating disorders such as bulimia and anorexia nervosa, and other conditions. Missed periods can be a warning sign that calcium is being lost from bones.

And, in any event, women are more likely candidates than men for osteoporosis because, most research shows, they start out with about 30 percent less bone mass, in proportion to body weight.

Q: Are there any other risk factors for osteoporosis?

A: There are several other major factors:

• Heredity. A family history of fractures; a small, slender body build; fair skin; and a Caucasian or Asian background can increase the risk for osteoporosis. Heredity also may help explain why some women develop osteoporosis early in life, even before they undergo menopause.

• Nutrition and lifestyle. Poor nutrition, including a diet that's low in calcium and vitamin D, and a sedentary lifestyle have been linked to osteoporosis. So have smoking and excessive alcohol consumption.

• Medications and other illnesses. Osteoporosis has been linked to some medications, including steroids, and to certain illnesses. For example, hyperthyroidism, or a chronically overactive thyroid gland, can decrease the calcium content of bones and accelerate the onset of osteoporosis.

Q: How can I tell if I have osteoporosis?

A: It often develops unnoticed over many years, with no symptoms or discomfort until a fracture occurs. As the condition progresses, however, one telltale sign is an excess **kyphosis**, or severely rounded upper back—better known as a ''dowager's hump.'' People with osteoporosis lose height, too, although that's also true of all people as they age and their discs absorb less water.

Q: But can a doctor test for osteoporosis?

A: If there isn't enough evidence, including X-rays, to confirm that you've got the condition, doctors can perform a diagnostic procedure called **bone densitometry**. It's a safe, painless X-ray technique that compares your bone density to the norm for a person of your age, gender and race. Often it's performed in women at the time of menopause to get a ''baseline'' bone-density measure.

If your doctor finds low bone mass, she may still want to perform additional tests to rule out the possibility of other diseases that can cause bone loss, such as osteomalacia, a vitamin D deficiency.

Q: What can I do to prevent osteoporosis?

A: You can't prevent it. Everyone eventually develops this condition, because everyone's bones become less dense over time. However, there is much you can do throughout your life to delay its development and protect yourself from fractures—mostly by "bone banking," or building up good bone mass before you age. You can do that by exercising, good nutrition and other healthy habits.

Q: I guess you mean a diet with plenty of calcium. Should I drink lots of milk?

A: Yes, or—given the fat content of milk—take calcium in some other form, including nonfat yogurt, calcium-rich foods such as broccoli and collard greens, and dietary supplements.

How much calcium you need depends on your age and other factors. The National Institutes of Health makes the following recommendations regarding daily intake of calcium:

- People ages 11 to 24 years: 1,200 milligrams
- Pregnant or nursing women under age 19: 2,000 mg.
- Pregnant or nursing women 19 years or older: 1,400 mg.
- Premenopausal women: 1,000 mg.
- Menopausal/postmenopausal women not taking estrogen: 1,500 mg.
- Menopausal/postmenopausal women taking estrogen: 1,000 mg.
- Middle-aged men: 1,000 mg.

To give you some guidance, we'll note that an eight-ounce glass of milk contains about 300 mg. of calcium.

Q: I can understand why calcium is needed for bones, but why do I need vitamin D? And how much do I need?

A: Vitamin D helps your body absorb calcium. The Food and Drug Administration recommends 400 I.U. (international units) daily. A cup of milk contains 100 I.U., so four cups of milk would take care of your calcium and vitamin D needs. If milk isn't your cup of tea, you can also get vitamin D from liver, egg yolks and fatty fish.

Alternatively, you can take vitamin supplements. But consult your doctor first, as vitamin D in excess can be toxic.

Q: Are there specific kinds of exercise that help fight osteoporosis?

A: To forestall and manage osteoporosis, the American Academy of Orthopaedic Surgeons (AAOS) recommends a program of moderate, regular exercise, three to four times a week. What's best are weight-bearing exercises, such as walking, jogging, hiking, climbing stairs, dancing, treadmill exercises and weight training—all of which help minimize bone loss.

"To help prevent bone loss," says Rebecca Jackson, M.D., associate professor of internal medicine at Ohio State University, in Columbus, "you need to do exercise that will create intermittent forces across the bone"—that is, force that comes and goes.

On a cautionary note, the AAOS suggests that, if you already have osteoporosis, you consult your doctor before embarking on an exercise program.

Q: Is there any evidence that exercise does actually strengthen bones?

A: Yes, there are a number of studies to that effect. Recently, for example, rcsearchers at Texas Woman's University, in Denton, found that young women enrolled in a 27-week gymnastics program increased the density of bone in their lower spine by 1.3 percent during the season. And the gymnasts, who had been exercising for an average of almost 10 years when they began the program, already had bones 8 to 10 percent denser than those of the women in the study who did not exercise.

Q: But what about more moderate exercises for older women? Is there proof they help?

A: Yes. Jackson and her colleagues recently studied the effectiveness of exercise on 14 sedentary women in their early 60s. Over the course of eight months, half the women took part in a three-times-a-week exercise program involving 30 minutes of stationary cycling; the second group had no exercise.

The researchers found that bone density in the spines of women in the exercise group increased, while it declined in the group that didn't exercise.

While the increase was modest, that rate of exercise over three years should increase bone density by 5 to 10 percent, a gain regarded as highly significant.

Q: What about other treatments? Isn't there special therapy for postmenopausal women?

A: **Estrogen replacement therapy (ERT)** is often recommended for menopausal or postmenopausal women who, based on bone-density measurements, are at high risk for osteoporosis. A study, which was led by Jane Cauley, Ph.D., at the University of Pittsburgh Graduate School of Public Health and published in the *Annals of Internal Medicine* in 1995, concluded that women who begin taking estrogen within five years of menopause and continue for the rest of their lives substantially decrease their risk of almost all fractures.

However, the study confirmed that, once you stop the therapy, your bone loss will return rapidly to its normal rate. That's why, before you undertake it, you should be aware that there are both good and bad side effects associated with the therapy, which is an area of active investigation by researchers.

Q: What are the side effects?

A: A recent and highly controversial Swedish study found that hormone replacement therapy may increase a woman's risk of breast cancer up to four times. Pending further research, such findings have kept a number of women from taking estrogen supplements.

In addition, estrogen, taken by itself, has been found to increase the risk of uterine cancer ninefold in postmenopausal women. To offset the uterine cancer risk, in recent years doctors have also prescribed a second hormone, progesterone. (The two hormones are combined in birth-control pills.) The downside was that the cardiovascular benefits that came from estrogen therapy then decreased.

However, a recent study found that estrogen in combination with progestin—a finely ground progesterone —restores the cardiovascular benefits without raising the risk of uterine cancer.

There was no evidence of an increased risk of breast cancer during the three years of the study, report Trudy Bush, Ph.D., of the University of Maryland School of Medicine, in Baltimore, and Elizabeth Barrett-Connor, Ph.D., of the University of California at San Diego.

Q: Does progestin have any adverse effects?

A: Progestin can trigger monthly bleeding, headaches, bloating and other symptoms similar to those of menstruation. On the plus side, the study did find that women taking hormone replacement therapy didn't gain as much weight after menopause as women taking no hormone therapy at all.

Q: Are there any other treatments for men and women with osteoporosis?

A: There are some medications, though they're still in the experimental stage. Doctors have found that large amounts of sodium fluoride—the compound added to drinking water to strengthen children's teeth—sometimes promotes the formation of bone. However, large quantities of fluoride can cause nausea, gastrointestinal bleeding and formation of bone spurs, contributing to stenosis, so it's a problematic therapy.

Other possible therapies include a thyroid hormone called calcitonin, which slows bone breakdown. However, it does not prevent fractures and must be injected three times weekly. Another is etidronate, a bisphosphonate drug that has been approved for Paget's disease. Ask your physician about them.

Further on the horizon is the possibility of gene therapy. Researchers have found that **osteoclasts**—the body's bone-destroying cells—produce large amounts of one enzyme found almost nowhere else in the body. They speculate that inhibiting this enzyme might halt the degeneration that occurs in osteoporosis.

Q: What if my bones are already brittle? Is there anything I can do to reduce the likelihood of fractures?

A: A study published in the *New England Journal of Medicine* in 1994 reported that elderly people can significantly reduce their risk of falling and thus their vulnerability to fractures.

Earlier studies had suggested that nothing could be done to prevent such falls, which are a major cause of death and disability. But the study, which was led by Mary Tinetti, M.D., of Yale University, found that people could avoid falls by monitoring blood pressure, taking prescription drugs carefully and learning ways to increase mobility. These included safer techniques for walking and getting out of the bath, and exercises to improve balance.

SPINAL CURVATURE

Q: What's wrong with spinal curvature? Don't all spines curve?

A: Absolutely. As we mentioned in Chapter 1, the normal spine has natural curves, apparent in a side view: a forward curve of the lumbar spine known as lordosis and a backward curve of the thoracic spine called kyphosis. The problem occurs when these curves become excessive.

Hyperlordosis, also known as excess lordosis or swayback, may be caused by a congenital defect—that is, one present at birth—or by a disease related to certain elements of the spine. Or it may be a postural problem, the result of trying to compensate for the imbalance of high heels or a large belly from pregnancy or obesity. In any event, the curve—by placing undue stress—can aggravate back pain in people who already have bulging discs or intervertebral facet-joint problems.

Excess kyphosis may develop in people with osteoporosis, as we mentioned earlier. But it can also occur in younger people as a result of muscle spasms or vertebral fractures in the low back. As the elderly population of the United States grows, the incidence of excess kyphosis is expected to increase, according to the AAOS.

Q: What's scoliosis?

A: Scoliosis—Greek for ''crookedness''—is a spinal curve that's side-to-side. In X-rays a scoliotic spine looks more like an ''S'' or a ''C'' than the straight line you see in a rear (not a side) view. Some of the bones in a scoliotic spine also may have rotated slightly, so that the person seems to be leaning to one side, and one hip appears higher than the other.

Q: Is it serious?

A: If untreated, it can either stabilize as a condition that's only a nuisance—skirts or trousers may need to be specially tailored so they hang evenly—or it may become much more serious. At its worse, it can lead to severe, early degenerative arthritis; chronic back pain; deformity; and—because of misshapen ribs—lung and heart disease that can shorten a person's life.

Q: Who gets scoliosis?

A: It affects about 2 percent of the population but it's much more common in some families; one theory is that there may be an inherited predisposition for asymmetrical, or unbalanced, growth. In any event, if someone in your family has scoliosis, the odds of your having it, too, are about 20 percent.

Generally scoliosis doesn't appear until the growth spurt of adolescence. It occurs in otherwise healthy children, and more often in girls than boys. In fact, some schools sponsor scoliosis screenings.

Since children with scoliosis aren't in pain, you've got to be alert for other signs. The American Academy of Orthopaedic Surgeons advises parents to watch for the following indications of scoliosis when their child is about eight years old:

- uneven shoulders
- prominent shoulder blade or blades
- uneven waist
- elevated hips
- leaning to one side

Q: Do adults ever develop scoliosis?

A: When adults seem to be developing scoliosis, it's generally a progression of a condition that began in childhood but went unnoticed. Sometimes, however, adult scoliosis can be caused by disc degeneration that occurs in an uneven pattern. Like excess kyphosis, it's expected that adult scoliosis will become more common as the population ages.

Q: How is scoliosis treated?

A: When children show early signs of scoliosis, physicians usually monitor it closely to ensure that it doesn't worsen. Most spinal curves in children remain minimal and don't require intervention. If the curvature does worsen, the doctor may recommend an orthopedic brace to prevent it from getting worse. If that doesn't control the curve or the scoliosis is already severe, surgery may be required. But that's relatively rare.

According to the AAOS, exercise and spinal manipulation are not effective against scoliosis. However, some doctors recommend exercise, and some chiropractors maintain that exercise alone can help stop scoliosis before it becomes a problem.

TUMORS

Q: Earlier you said that cancer can cause back pain. So if I don't know why my back hurts, should I worry about a tumor?

A: You can worry about it, but it's a rare event. In *Your Aching Back,* Augustus White estimates that "probably fewer than one in 10,000 backache patients has cancer in the spine." Having said that, we'll note that tumors can affect any of the spine's structures—the bone, ligaments, nerves, muscles or synovial tissue—and that a backache can be a primary symptom.

Q: What kinds of tumors attack the spine?

A: There are primary tumors, which originate in the spine and may be either malignant or benign, and metastatic tumors, which spread to the spine from malignancies in other parts of the body. These secondary tumors of the spine are more common than primary tumors.

Malignant tumors of the spine include **multiple myelomas**, which attack the bone marrow in many parts of the body; tumors of the lymph system; and **schwannomas** and **neurofibromas**, which arise from the nerve roots. Benign tumors include

osteoid osteoma, a bony tumor that causes severe back pain; and **meningioma**, which is found in the thoracic spine or the spinal canal.

Q: What are some of the cancers that metastasize to the spine?

A: Breast, lung and prostate cancers—the latter a problem afflicting mainly older men—are the most common sources of spinal metastases as well as the most common cancers in general. Thyroid, intestinal and kidney tumors also metastasize to the spine.

In addition, experts suggest that young men with back pain should be examined for testicular cancer. In some cases, back pain is the first symptom of testicular cancer, even when the cancer has not spread to the spine.

Q: How would I suspect that cancer—rather than, say, arthritis—might be causing my back pain?

A: If it's a metastatic tumor, you'd probably have had symptoms elsewhere that would have sent you to a doctor before you developed back pain. And since such tumors tend to metastasize to other locations before the spine, you'd have plenty of warning.

Moreover, back pain from a tumor is noticeably different from pain caused by a ruptured disc, for example. It tends to be continuous. Bed rest doesn't provide any relief and, particularly if the tumor is malignant, the pain gets steadily worse.

If the tumor grows unimpeded, it may cause spinal-cord compression that gets progressively worse over months or even years. In addition to back pain, you may develop stiff legs, a diminished sense of where your feet or toes are, and problems with bladder or bowel function.

Q: Aren't there any tests for spinal tumors?

A: Tumors are usually diagnosed by a thorough examination combined with X-rays, an MRI, CT scan, a myelogram of the spine or a **bone scan**—the latter a procedure in which a radioactive material, injected into the bloodstream, settles into the bones and reveals areas that are undergoing rapid cell growth. If your doctor does find a tumor, he'd perform a biopsy to determine whether it was benign or malignant, and proceed from there with surgery, radiation and/or chemotherapy.

INFECTIONS

Q: You said infections can also cause back pain. How does a spine get infected?

A: The spine can become infected through a number of routes: an open fracture or wound (including a surgical incision) that exposes the bone; a simple boil on the skin or gum disease that spreads bacteria through the bloodstream; the use of unsterile needles by drug addicts. Additionally, tuberculosis, infections of the urinary tract from indwelling urinary catheters, and kidney infections can all travel to spine.

Keep in mind that these are very rare, particularly with the advent of antibiotics and other modern medicines. However, if you're diabetic, you do run a higher risk because your resistance to infection is lower.

Q: What kinds of infections are there?

A: There are infections of the vertebrae, the connective tissues (including discs) and even—in the case of **meningitis**—the membrane that covers the spinal cord. There are also abscesses that occur in the epidural space, which is the space between the covering of the spinal cord and the outer covering of the vertebral column.

Arguably the most common spinal infection is **vertebral osteomyelitis**, an infection of the vertebral body that occurs through the routes mentioned above. Less understood is a condition called **discitis**, in which one or two discs of the lumbar spine become inflamed and extremely painful. While some experts believe discitis is an infection, others think it's simply an inflammatory response. Discitis tends to occur in younger people, under the age of 20.

Q: How can I tell when I've got a spinal infection?

A: A recent history of urinary tract infection, surgery or intravenous drug use is usually a giveaway. Another telltale sign is that, in addition to severe and unrelenting back pain, you may have fever or chills. People with meningitis typically have a high fever, headache and a stiff neck as well as back pain.

In other cases, a spinal infection shows up as referred pain: A man with a cervical spine infection may say his head hurts, or a woman with a thoracic infection thinks she's having a heart attack. According to Martin C. McHenry, M.D., an infectious disease specialist at the Cleveland Clinic, it's not unknown for people with lower-thoracic or upper-lumbar spinal infections to undergo an unnecessary appendectomy or gall bladder surgery.

Q: How are infections diagnosed?

A: An elevated sedimentation rate suggests infection, and a variety of imaging techniques —X-rays, CT scans, myelograms—may confirm the diagnosis. However, particularly in the early stages, an infection such as vertebral osteomyelitis is hard to detect by X-ray. Once it is suspected, doctors will perform a needle biopsy to diagnose which bacteria is causing the problem.

Q: Can these spinal infections be treated?

A: They can be treated effectively with antibiotics, if they're bacterial infections. For disc infections, doctors sometimes immobilize patients with a body cast or a brace, and for discitis steroids like cortisone have been prescribed. In some cases, surgery may be necessary.

Left untreated, spinal infections can become quite serious, causing damage to the vertebrae that may require a long recovery period or even resulting in neurological damage or death.

OTHER BACK DISORDERS

Q: Are there any other back conditions that cause back pain?

A: There are several less common conditions that deserve some attention, including **fibrositis**, **spondylolytic** conditions and **syringomyelia**. We'll start at the bottom, with **coccydynia**, or coccygeal pain.

Q: Coccygeal pain? That involves the coccyx, right?

A: That's right. One of the most common causes of coccygeal pain is a hard fall on the tailbone, usually on the floor or the stairs. But the coccyx can also become irritated in some people simply because it's the focus of pressure in a sitting position. And sometimes the pain is related to psychological stress.

Q: How is it treated?

A: Usually by removing pressure on the coccyx. You might try sitting on a cushion that displaces some of the body's weight onto the buttocks and legs.

Stephen Hochschuler of the Texas Back Institute recommends treating it with anti-inflammatory medicine or, if that doesn't work, an injection of cortisone around the coccyx.

Q: What are the spondylolytic conditions you mentioned?

A: The first, which is called **spondylolysis**, is an anatomic gap in the back of a vertebra in the low back, due to vertebral defects, or cracks. Gymnasts and other athletes who do a lot of hyperextension—back arching—tend to develop these "fatigue breaks" or "stress fractures" in the bone.

Some people have this condition and never develop symptoms. In others, it can lead to **spondylolisthesis**.

Q: What's that?

A: Literally, it's "slipping vertebrae." It's a condition in which, as the name suggests, a defect or crack in a vertebra allows it to slip forward, forcing the spine out of alignment and causing several vertebrae above that one to slide forward, too. Usually it occurs in the lower lumbar spine, just above the sacrum, or at L4/L5.

Q: Who gets spondylolisthesis?

A: The condition affects as much as 2 to 3 percent of the population and, as you'd suspect, it includes a disproportionate number of athletes—particularly those who do a lot of flexion and extension of the low back and subject those vertebrae to repeated stress. According to Augustus White, spondylolisthesis is four times more common in football players than in the general population.

For the record, the other group that has a predisposition for spondylolisthesis is Eskimos.

Q: How can I tell if I've got a spondylolytic condition?

A: Symptoms include severe low-back pain, pain in the hips and thighs and, if there's nerve root irritation, sciatica. You may have tight hamstring muscles and a stiff-legged walk.

Your personal history—if you're an athlete, or do a lot of heavy lifting—would raise your doctor's suspicions, and she can confirm the diagnosis with plain X-rays or a bone scan.

Q: How are spondylolytic conditions treated?

A: Initially, with rest, painkillers and braces. Lyle J. Micheli, M.D., an orthopedic surgeon at Harvard Medical School, says he puts patients in a lumbosacral brace for six months, 23 hours a day.

During their free hours, they bathe and do exercises to strengthen their backs and make their spines more flexible.

If that doesn't work, surgery may be advised.

Q: What's fibrositis?

A: Fibrositis, or inflammation of the fibrous tissue —also known as fibromyalgia (pain in the muscle and fascia, the fibrous tissue covering it) or myofascial pain—is one of the more elusive sources of back pain. The condition, which typically occurs in middle-aged women, is often misdiagnosed as arthritis because its symptoms include an all-over achiness, pains and stiffness, often of many joints. But unlike arthritis, fibrositis is characterized by so-called trigger points or tender points—points in the body that are very tender to the touch.

Fibrositis is also distinguished by what's known as nonrestorative sleep; people with the condition wake up tired after a full night's sleep. Sleep researchers have found that people who have this syndrome have a peculiar brain-sleep-wave pattern, as though they were awake and asleep at the same time.

Q: How is it treated?

A: Some doctors prescribe low dosages of an antidepressant like amitriptyline (Elavil, made by Roche), not because the person is depressed, but because it changes her brain chemistry so that she can sleep deeply. In addition to Elavil, people may be helped by injections at the trigger points with local anesthetic or an acupuncture needle, or by anesthetic spray, massage, manipulation or low-impact exercise.

Q: Are there any other conditions that cause back pain?

A: There's a neurological disease called syringomyelia in which cysts form inside the spinal cord. The cysts press against nerves, causing numbness and sometimes irreversible damage. It's believed that the disease is caused by a developmental malformation of the cerebellum that allows spinal fluid to seep into the spinal cord and form cysts. The principal treatment is surgery to rechannel the spinal fluid outside the spinal cord.

Q: How common is syringomyelia?

A: That's hard to say. Traditionally it's been regarded as a so-called orphan disease—by definition, a disease affecting no more than 200,000 people. However, some sufferers and their physicians are convinced that, because the disease can be readily diagnosed only by MRI, many cases of syringomyelia have been passed off as chronic back pain.

REFERRED BACK PAIN

Q: You said earlier that some conditions can cause back pain without actually involving the back. What are they?

A: There are many: diseases of the abdomen and pelvic region, including acute prostatitis, or inflammation of the prostate; diseases of the large intestine, such as inflammation, ulcers or tumors; bladder and kidney diseases, particularly an infection or kidney stone; and arthritis, infections or tumors of the hip area.

In each case, usually other symptoms indicate that the back pain is only referred. If the pain is caused by an ulcer, for example, it's likely to surface shortly after eating and to be soothed by certain foods. Kidney disease and prostatitis also produce urinary problems. And as a rule, rest or activity has no effect on the pain.

Q: Doesn't menstruation often cause back pain?

A: Yes, many women develop back pain when they're either menstruating or in midcycle. In fact, a number of gynecological disorders—infected fallopian tubes, a prolapsed or tipped uterus, endometriosis and tumors of the reproductive organs—can produce deep pain in the low back.

Q: Are there any other major sources of referred pain?

A: Vascular disease, such as an arteriosclerosis that blocks arteries carrying blood to the legs, can produce symptoms that are sometimes blamed on spinal stenosis; there's back and leg pain that gets worse with walking, and a pins-and-needles tingling in the legs. People can also get sudden back pain from an aortic aneurysm, the ballooning of the main artery from the heart—a life-threatening condition for which, in contrast to the vast majority of genuine back problems, surgery may be unavoidable.

4 SURGERY

Q: What conditions require back surgery?

A: Surgery may be performed when conservative treatment is ineffective for alleviating disc problems as well as many of the conditions described in Chapter 3.

Basically, there are two main types of back operations: **decompression**, involving the removal of pressure on the nerves in the spinal canal caused by a herniated disc; and **fusion**, which involves fusing two or more vertebrae together to stabilize the spine and thus prevent any painful movement.

There are varied procedures within each of these categories, and some operations may involve both categories. In addition, there are a few types of operations —notably nervous-system surgery and surgery to treat spinal infections—that don't fit into either category.

In this chapter, we'll describe the most common types of back operations.

Q: How frequently is surgery performed?

A: In 1994, according to an estimate by the Texas Back Institute, about 250,000 people had a **discectomy**. This is the most common back operation, and involves the removal of all or part of a herniated disc. That compares with about 200,000 in previous years.

Q: Why is it increasing?

A: Richard A. Deyo, M.D., a leading orthopedic researcher, suggests that the increase may be due in part to the availability of improved imaging techniques, such as MRI, which are capable of detecting partially herniated discs that otherwise would go unnoticed. However, as we indicated earlier, many of the ruptures that show up on MRIs aren't causing pain and should be ignored.

Q: You mean there's too much back surgery?

A: Increasingly, many leading back-care experts in various specialties believe there's too much back surgery. Stephen Hochschuler of the Texas Back Institute says emphatically, "Half of all back surgeries performed in the United States are unnecessary."

There is substantially more back surgery in the United States than in countries, such as Canada, with national health programs that limit physicians' fees. "There are almost 20 times more back operations per capita in the

United States than Canada," David Imrie, M.D., director of the Back Power Program, a rehabilitation clinic in Toronto, told *American Health* magazine a few years ago. "And it isn't because the results are so good. Surgery is definitely overdone."

Admittedly, such statements are based on clinical experience and observation, not on research. And it could be argued that many back conditions that should be treated surgically get short shrift in countries with national health programs.

Q: How successful is back surgery?

A: The success rate of back surgery varies considerably with the particular procedure, from an excellent 90-percent-or-so rate of success to rates that are pretty unacceptable. But, like back problems, success in back surgery is often hard to define. Many patients whose surgery is deemed successful are disappointed by their postoperative condition, which may include residual pain and limited mobility and flexibility.

Q: Is there a way of improving the success rate?

A: Obviously, get a good surgeon—one who not only has a good technique but recognizes what's operable and what isn't. You might think that is stating the obvious, but as Richard Fraser, M.D., a professor of neurosurgery at Cornell University Medical College, puts it succinctly, "Failed back surgery is usually due to operating on the wrong patient."

Q: How can doctors be sure whether or not I should have surgery?

A: Hamilton Hall, M.D., an orthopedic surgeon who is on staff at the Orthopaedic and Arthritic Hospital, in Toronto, Canada, uses this rule in his book, *More Advice From the Back Doctor:* "A back problem must be structural, localized and specific—an unstable joint or pressure on a nerve root."

According to David Borenstein, M.D., of the George Washington University Medical Center, in Washington, D.C., "The need for lumbar spine surgery is limited to 1 to 2 percent of individuals in whom conservative management has failed." Borenstein says the people with the best chance of successful surgery are those whose clinical symptoms, physical exam findings and imaging studies all corroborate which structure is causing the problem.

Q: What about complications?

A: There are a number of potential complications, related to the specific nature of back surgery and the nature of surgery generally. Back surgery can be a physically traumatic procedure requiring a large incision, lengthy hospital stay and extended recovery. The close proximity of the spinal structures to the main highway of nerves has made it difficult to introduce any technique that might restrict the surgeon's view, so until recently surgeons have traditionally fully exposed the spine at the affected site.

And even so, surgeons may get it wrong. According to Fraser, "The most common error in back surgery is operating on the wrong level of the spine"—usually the wrong lumbar disc.

Any surgery has risks, mainly from infection. But the risk most feared by the public in back surgery, according to the American Medical Association (AMA), is paralysis —and that's largely unwarranted. Most back surgery is performed on the low back, leaving a comfortable margin of safety between the operating site and the spinal cord. Cervical spine surgery does carry a risk of general paralysis but, according to the AMA, it's less than one per 1,000.

We'll talk more about specific risks later in this chapter.

Q: Who should perform the surgery?

A: An Australian study found that orthopedic surgeons and neurosurgeons had about the same success rate for low-back discectomies. However, Augustus White, a leading orthopedic surgeon at Harvard Medical School, says spinal fusions are best left to orthopedic surgeons, who are generally more experienced. And neurosurgeons typically perform the nervous-system operations described at the end of this chapter.

DISCECTOMIES

Q: What's involved in a discectomy?

A: There are several different approaches, all with the goal of decompression, or removing that part of the disc that's pressing on nerves.

For the past 50 years, the standard procedure has been a **laminectomy** with discectomy, which involves removing the **lamina**—the bony plate on the back of the vertebrae—as well as part of the disc. In recent years technology has brought dramatic change to back surgery through such procedures as the **microdiscectomy** and the **percutaneous discectomy**. We'll describe them all in this section.

Keep in mind that, while there are cervical discectomies, in most cases we're talking about procedures involving lumbar discs—typically L4/L5 or L5/S1.

Q: Let's take the procedures one at a time. What happens in a laminectomy with discectomy?

A: The surgeon, using X-rays to pinpoint the problem disc, makes a two-inch incision (or longer, if more than one disc is involved) in the back. He cuts out the entire lamina (if only a portion of lamina is removed, the procedure is called a **laminotomy**) as well as part of the ligament, creating an opening into the spinal canal. Carefully moving aside the bundle of nerves called the cauda equina, he then exposes the disc.

What the surgeon does next depends on the condition of the disc. If there's a detached or ''free'' fragment of disc in the canal, he simply removes it. If the disc is extruding or protruding, however—conditions we described in Chapter 2—the surgeon removes the bulging part as well as some disc material that may become a problem in the future.

Q: How much of the disc is removed?

A: Most surgeons remove only the part of the disc that is causing the trouble, and a bit beyond that. "This usually means taking all of the extruded part of the disc and perhaps 20 percent of the remainder," White says in *Your Aching Back.* The goal is to leave enough of the disc to provide shock absorbency between vertebrae, while removing enough to minimize the likelihood that it will herniate again.

Q: If all (or most) of the disc is removed, won't the vertebrae scrape together?

A: No, but occasionally the spine may become so unstable that it becomes necessary to fuse two vertebrae together. This involves the process known as spinal fusion, which we discuss later in this chapter.

Q: Can an artificial disc be inserted?

A: There have been efforts for years to develop something to replace a problem disc, but one problem has been finding an appropriate material that's strong enough to last 40 or 50 years. A team of scientists at the Johns Hopkins Medical School, led by orthopedic surgeon John Kostuik, has developed a disc made of titanium and cobalt chrome, but they're still awaiting approval from the Food and Drug Administration to begin testing it in people.

Q: Is the discectomy a successful procedure?

A: That depends partly on the surgeon's skill, as you might suspect, and partly on some surprising factors, like the degree of disc deterioration. According to White, there's a 90 percent chance that the operation will relieve sciatica if the disc has completely ruptured. If the disc has only extruded, he says, the success rate drops to 80 percent. And if the disc was only bulging, success is in the range of 60 percent.

While those are still fairly decent odds, some research suggests that a discectomy is no more or less effective than nonsurgical treatment. According to the federal panel on low-back pain, "With or without surgery, 80 percent of patients with sciatica recover eventually." A Swedish study of people with herniated discs found that, while surgical patients returned to work sooner, six months after treatment there was little difference between those who had had discectomies and those who opted for nonsurgical treatment with immobilization. However, the surgical patients rated their condition as more improved.

Other studies from Norway show that surgical patients were better for two to five years but, after 10 years, patients who hadn't had surgery were doing just as well.

Q: You mentioned microdiscectomy. What's that?

A: It's essentially the same procedure, but performed through an operating microscope that greatly magnifies the surgical field. It allows the surgeon not only to make a smaller incision but also to remove less muscle from the spine in order to enter the spinal canal. Also, postoperative recovery is easier; the procedure may even be performed on an outpatient basis.

Q: It sounds a lot better than the traditional discectomy. Why isn't it used all the time?

A: There are disadvantages to this approach. While it may be ideal for plucking out detached or free fragments, the limited access makes it harder to remove all the other problematic disc material.

So the procedure gets mixed reviews. Fraser of Cornell says that, in the hands of an experienced surgeon who selects appropriate patients, "the benefits [of microdiscectomy] generally outweigh the risks." On the other hand, White endorses the traditional "open" approach.

Q: What's a percutaneous discectomy?

A: It's a procedure in which part of the offending disc is removed with suction. The surgeon makes a tiny incision (about a quarter-inch) in the skin and, guided by a X-ray machine, inserts a hollow probe up to the annulus of the problem disc. With a second instrument, he then cuts and suctions out small pieces of disc. When percutaneous discectomy was introduced, it was done manually. Now, however, surgeons perform automated percutaneous discectomy, in which a probe —operated with a foot pedal—automatically cuts and sucks away the tissue.

Q: What's the recovery period like?

A: Percutaneous discectomy, which takes 45 minutes and is carried out under local anesthetic, may be performed on an outpatient basis, and patients may return to activity a week later.

Obviously that compares favorably with a traditional "open" discectomy, which requires general anesthesia, three or four days in the hospital and a six-week recovery period.

Q: If I must have disc surgery, percutaneous discectomy sounds like the way to go. Why isn't it done all the time?

A: It isn't suitable for everyone—in fact, it isn't suitable at all for free fragments, the condition that benefits most from traditional discectomies. However, the main drawback seems to be that the procedure is still comparatively new and untested, and there are no long-term studies establishing its safety or efficacy. In his book, *The Well-Informed Patient's Guide to Back Surgery,* Fraser says, "many back surgeons believe percutaneous discectomy is neither as predictable nor as successful as either standard laminectomy/discectomy or microsurgical discectomy." In fact, the federal panel on acute low-back pain found percutaneous discectomy significantly less effective than even chemonucleolysis, the problematic nonsurgical disc procedure described in Chapter 2.

Q: Are there any other ways to operate on discs?

A: Arthroscopic surgery, which has been used for knee and other joint operations for some time, has been tried recently for herniated discs. In it, surgeons insert an **arthroscope**, a flexible viewing tube that contains optical fibers, a small lens and a light scope, through a small incision into the disc, to look directly at the disc material being removed. The view can be magnified and displayed on a video screen.

Q: Is arthroscopic surgery used much for discs?

A: The area where it's making the biggest impact, in back surgery, is on thoracic discs. Until recently, the only way to reach a herniated thoracic disc was a complex procedure called a **thoracotomy**, which involved an eight-inch incision reaching from the center of the patient's chest, across the rib cage and around to the midback. The surgeon had to spread the rib cage, stretch nerve tissue, and cut shoulder muscle to reach the thoracic spine.

Even as back surgery goes, it's an extremely sensitive procedure, coming right up against the spinal cord. About a quarter of patients suffer "post-thoracotomy pain syndrome," persistent discomfort from the stretching of nerves, and the recovery period may be three months.

Q: What's changed as a result of the arthroscope?

A: With **video-assisted thoracoscopy (VAT)**, the surgeon makes a few small incisions through which he inserts one tube that lights the area and transmits video to television monitors, and other tubes that cut and suction the disc material. Patients leave the hospital after two days, and return to activity within a month.

Recently VAT has been used for numerous thoracic spine problems, including tumors, infections and deformities such as scoliosis as well as herniated discs. ''As we develop this procedure and further refine the instruments, it is conceivable that 90 percent of thoracic spine surgeries can be done this way,'' says Texas Back Institute spine surgeon John Regan, M.D.

Q: What's the procedure for a herniated cervical disc?

A: For the most part, neck-disc surgery is similar to back-disc surgery. However, some surgeons prefer to make their incision in the front of the neck, rather than the back. Also, because the neck is more flexible than the low back and the frontal approach removes a large amount of the nucleus of the disc, the procedure will probably be combined with a spinal fusion.

Q: Who has discectomies?

A: According to a study several years ago, the average age of a patient undergoing lumbar discectomy is 38 years. The same study found that men are almost twice as likely as women to have a discectomy for a herniated lumbar disc.

Since epidemiological studies indicate that men are only slightly more prone to herniated discs than women, we can only speculate on the reasons for the difference in surgical rates. It could be that many orthopedists follow White's practice in urging prompt disc surgery for two groups of individuals who can't wait to see if time will heal: professional athletes and workers with strenuous lifting tasks.

Q: You said that surgery for a herniated disc is the most common back operation. When should I have surgery?

A: Before they operate, leading orthopedists say they require the following conditions:

- A clear image of herniation on an MRI or CT scan
- Physical evidence, such as the straight-leg-raising test, and pain that corresponds to the disc herniation
- Evidence such as an electromyographic study that identifies nerve root damage by an encroaching disc
- Failure to respond to at least four to six weeks of nonsurgical therapy

Q: Is it okay to delay surgery longer than that?

A: Timing can be an important issue. Back surgery isn't something you want to rush into, but if it's inevitable, it's not something you want to postpone too long, either.

Doctors usually tell patients to wait six weeks to determine whether the pain has subsided or whether surgery is warranted, according to the American Academy of Orthopaedic Surgeons (AAOS). But six weeks seems to be a make-or-break point, too: If you are going to have elective disc surgery, the ideal time is at about six weeks after you first develop leg pain.

In *Your Aching Back,* White writes that "the best information suggests that herniated-disc patients who wait less than 60 days have a better surgical prognosis than those who wait longer. If you're going to have elective disc surgery, the ideal time is at about 40 to 50 days (six weeks) after the onset of leg pain.

"Patients who undergo disc removal after being laid up for a year are only half as likely to get pain relief as patients who have surgery earlier," writes White, adding that the same is true for mobility. "If one watches a 'foot drop' motor weakness too long—more than three, six or nine months—it may not recover for one to two years after surgery, if at all."

Q: Why is it bad to delay surgery beyond a certain point?

A: It's not clear. It may be that, as time goes by, the nerve roots become irreparably scarred by compression and inflammation. White speculates there may be a psychological factor: People who become accustomed to chronic pain can't easily forget it, even when the cause has disappeared.

Q: Is there such a thing as emergency back surgery?

A: Yes, when someone has cauda equina syndrome, the condition described in Chapter 2. Unless it's corrected promptly with a discectomy, the person may be left with permanent incontinence.

SPINAL FUSION

Q: So a spinal fusion is performed after disc surgery? When else?

A: In fact, fusions aren't performed that frequently with a simple lumbar discectomy. More often they're performed because of severe arthritis—worn facet joints or degenerative discs—or when vertebrae have been seriously damaged, as in an accident, for example.

Fusions may also be performed in conjunction with some of the conditions discussed in the previous chapter: spinal stenosis, scoliosis and spondylolisthesis, in which vertebrae tend to slip out of alignment. A survey of athletic patients with spondylolysis—a related condition described in Chapter 3—found that nearly 10 percent required fusion surgery.

Q: What actually takes place in a spinal fusion?

A: In a simple fusion procedure, the surgeon makes an incision—usually in the back, but sometimes in the abdomen—about three inches long and, as in a discectomy, pushes aside muscles and ligaments to reach the vertebrae. He attaches bone grafts, about the size and shape of matchsticks, onto the facet joints. Larger pieces of bone are used between vertebrae.

Over time—generally four to nine months—the bones and bone grafts grow together, and the two vertebrae are fused into a single, solid unit.

Q: Where do these bone grafts come from?

A: They're usually from either the patient himself—sliced off the pelvis during the same operation—or a "bone bank" such as that operated by the American Red Cross. A third possibility is animal bone, which is considered almost, but not quite, as effective as human bank bone.

Q: Which is better, donated bone or my own?

A: Both have pros and cons. If you use your own, you're subjecting yourself to a second incision and an additional risk of infection or a hematoma, a localized collection of blood in the tissues.

On the other hand, your own bone won't be rejected by your body and—unlike bank bone—it may stimulate new bone growth. In addition, bank bone carries a minuscule risk of transmitting a blood-borne disease such as hepatitis, syphilis or AIDS. According to Augustus White, there's been one documented case in which a patient contracted AIDS as a result of a bone graft used in a spinal fusion. The bone was donated by someone who had AIDS.

If the bank bone—known as an **allograph**—is obtained and managed according to the American Association of Tissue Banks' standards, the risk of AIDS is virtually eliminated.

Q: **What's the success rate?**

A: An unremarkable 60 to 70 percent overall, according to Augustus White; as he notes, that isn't much better than rates for a variety of nonoperative treatments described in Chapter 2. That rate reflects both pain and mobility; the federal panel on acute low-back pain noted that there is no good evidence that patients who undergo fusion will return to their prior functional level.

However, when fusion is done for scoliosis, spondylolisthesis and certain other conditions, the odds are much better. According to Scott Blumenthal, M.D., of the Texas Back Institute, fusion is successful about 80 percent of the time in relieving the severe back and leg pain often caused by spondylolisthesis.

Q: Is it a risky procedure?

A: There's always the risk of wound infections, as well as chronic pain where the bone graft was removed. There's the additional risk of **pseudarthrosis**, a condition in which all or part of a fusion fails to take, leaving the back painful and unstable. This can be corrected by further surgery, as we discuss in the next section.

Q: Aren't metal implants or pins ever used in a fusion?

A: Various types of implants—rods, wires, hooks and screws—may be used to secure the vertebrae for several months after surgery, fusing with the bone graft as it heals. They're used most in operations for scoliosis, and seem to help the most when there are fusions involving three or more vertebrae.

Q: Are there risks from these implants?

A: Yes, although the precise degree of risk is debatable. Recently Public Citizen, a Washington, D.C., consumer advocacy group, asked the Food and Drug Administration (FDA) to stop allowing the use of steel screw implants in people's spines as a treatment for back pain.

The group argued that they cause complications ranging from infection to leg weakness and paralysis (from nerve damage) in one-third of all patients. Public

Citizen also said screw recipients are twice as likely to need additional spinal operations as patients who undergo traditional spinal fusions without screws.

The FDA said it was aware of the complications but added that the screws are beneficial for people with fractures and severe spinal degeneration.

OTHER TYPES OF BACK SURGERY

Q: What other types of operations are performed on the back?

A: There are several other operations specifically for some of the conditions we discussed in Chapter 3, including spinal stenosis, ankylosing spondylitis, tumors and infection. And when all else fails, there's nervous-system surgery to alleviate back and leg pain.

Q: Let's start with spinal stenosis. What's the procedure?

A: Like the laminectomy with discectomy, this is a decompression procedure to relieve pressure on the spinal cord. In fact, the typical operation for spinal stenosis is known as a multiple laminectomy. It may also involve spinal fusion.

Usually the operation centers on the middle of the low back, and the surgeon may work up and down from there. The surgeon opens the spinal column at the specific points where it's narrowed, and then removes the bone or fibrous tissue—enlarged facet joints, ligaments and spinous process as well as lamina—that are pushing against the spinal cord. He may enlarge the openings through which the spinal nerve roots pass and, infrequently, remove a disc or disc fragments.

If an extensive amount of bone is removed, two or more vertebrae may need to be fused together to stabilize the spinal column.

Q: What are the odds that surgery for spinal stenosis will be successful?

A: They're excellent—an 80 to 90 percent chance of significant improvement or, at the very least, that your condition won't get worse, according to various studies.

For many people, the improvement is immediate: They can stand on the day surgery is performed and, by the time they leave the hospital a week or so later, they probably have less leg pain than when they arrived, various orthopedists say. Experts caution, however, that while decompression will relieve leg pain, it won't improve the back pain associated with disc deterioration, which will continue to take place.

Q: What's the operation for ankylosing spondylitis?

A: When ankylosing spondylitis becomes so severe that an individual is virtually doubled over, surgeons sometimes perform a procedure called an **osteotomy** to straighten the spine. They cut across the fused bone, surgically fracturing the spine and removing a wedge of bone.

Q: It sounds dangerous—is it?

A: It's quite dangerous, with one in every 10 or 20 patients dying or suffering major complications, according to Augustus White. One reason is that the procedure is done close to the spinal cord; another is that people who need this operation are already debilitated, with poor heart and lung function.

Q: You said earlier that there are operations for spinal infections. Why would they require surgery?

A: If the infection doesn't respond to antibiotics, it may be necessary to perform an operation called a **debridement**, in which the infected area is cleaned and pus, dead bone and foreign particles are washed out with antibiotic solutions. Because it may be necessary to remove enough bone to cure the infection, the surgeon may then have to perform a fusion.

Q: What about spinal tumors? How do doctors choose between surgery and chemotherapy or radiation?

A: Doctors are more likely to opt first for surgery if the tumor is primary—meaning that it originated in the back rather than spreading to it from the breast, for example—and if it's malignant, not benign. They may prefer radiation or chemotherapy for metastatic tumors. However, surgery may also be recommended if it's a metastatic tumor that's growing close to the nerves or becoming extremely painful due to movement of the spine.

The surgeon typically performs a multiple laminectomy to remove all the tumor plus a margin of normal spine. If a lot of spinc is removed, she may need to perform spinal reconstruction.

Q: What's involved in spinal reconstruction?

A: The spine may be rebuilt with a combination of bone graft, metal and even a **prosthesis** made of polymethylacrylate, a cement used in total joint replacement as well as spine surgery. This is a rare procedure and requires great surgical expertise.

Q: You mentioned nervous-system surgery. What's involved?

A: It's a type of surgery that may be used when all else fails—an example of what's known in the trade as "salvage surgery." In general, it involves cutting the nerves that transmit pain messages to the spinal cord and brain from areas such as the back or the legs.

One example of such surgery is a procedure called a **rhizotomy**, or rhizolysis, in which the surgeon tries to alleviate facet-joint pain by cauterizing, or searing, the tissues around the joints—thus destroying the nerves contained in those tissues.

Another example is a **cordotomy**, or tractotomy, a procedure most often used for cancer patients whose pain is excruciating and highly localized. In a cordotomy, the surgeon makes an incision to reach the spinal cord and then divides the spino-thalamic tract, which conducts pain from the body to the brain.

Q: What are the results of such procedures?

A: Immediate, but usually temporary, pain relief. In both cases, according to Richard Fraser, the pain may come back worse than before, partly because the nerves regenerate and partly because they're scarred and inflamed from the surgery. Furthermore, people who have a cordotomy run a risk of losing their motor control and may become incontinent.

As a result, this type of surgery is reserved mainly for people with terminal cancer. And even for them, other pain-control methods, such as a continuous infusion of morphine, are tried first.

Q: You mentioned salvage surgery. Is it all as dreadful as it sounds?

A: Salvage surgery is an appropriately alarming term to describe an alarming situation: the case of an individual who's had two or more back operations and has returned for another. The prognosis for such people is appalling. According to Augustus White, the chances of success are 30 percent for a second operation, 25 percent for a third, and 5 percent for a fourth —roughly the same as the chances that it will make the situation worse, as trauma to the nerves and muscles from surgery, and the formation of scar tissue cause more pain and disability.

It's not altogether clear why these odds are so dismal. However, one likely explanation—as we indicated early in this chapter—is that the initial surgery wasn't the correct course. To repeat the words of Richard Fraser, "Failed back surgery is usually due to operating on the wrong patient."

Q: Is repeat surgery ever justified?

A: Yes, mostly if the back surgery is for a completely different condition. A second or even third operation may be advisable if, after the first surgery: spinal stenosis develops (due to scarring or overgrowth of a fusion) or recurs; or the same or another disc herniates; or the patient develops pseudarthrosis. Finally, if the patient has had unsuccessful back surgery but not fusion, he may benefit from a spinal fusion.

It's been shown that repeat surgery is most likely to succeed when the patient has been free of pain for at least six months after the first operation.

5 PREVENTION

Q: How can I prevent back problems?

A: There are a great many things you can do, simply by modifying your lifestyle and daily habits, that can prevent you from getting back pain in the first place or, if you've had a bad back, suffering a recurrence.

As we've indicated in previous chapters, physical fitness is critical to a healthy back. In fact, heredity aside, it may be the most important factor. That means controlling your diet to avoid obesity, and quitting or reducing smoking. Exercise is essential to any back-pain prevention program; at the same time, there are certain sports that may be harmful to your back.

In addition, ergonomics has provided us with guidance concerning virtually every aspect of movement (or even nonmovement) that involves your back at work or play, from sitting and standing to lifting heavy objects. We discuss those at length in this chapter.

Q: Smoking? Sure, I know it's bad for my lungs—but my back?

A: Although there's no definitive relationship, several reports and studies in recent years have suggested that smokers are more likely to suffer disc damage, and that their discs are less likely to heal. One theory is that smokers often develop a chronic cough that increases pressure on the discs.

But most experts believe that smoking reduces the blood flow to the vertebrae and around the discs. "Anything that affects the blood supply to other parts of the body probably affects the spine as well," says Thomas E. Williamson-Kirkland, M.D., of the department of physical medicine and rehabilitation at Virginia Mason Medical Center.

Q: Exactly how risky is smoking?

A: According to a recent study by Howard An, M.D., of the Medical College of Wisconsin, smoking a pack or more a day quadrupled the risk of a serious disc problem in the neck and tripled the risk for low-back disc problems. The good news is that, if you quit now, your risk in five years will match that of nonsmokers, according to An.

Q: I know I should watch my weight. But is there anything in particular I should eat for a healthy back?

A: Good nutrition is good for your back as well as your general well-being, so be sure you have a diet with the proper balance of proteins, carbohydrates, fats, vitamins, minerals and water. As we mentioned in Chapter 3, calcium and vitamin D help build and strengthen bone.

Vitamin C helps in the formation of collagen, the connective tissue in bones, cartilage and skin, and is very important in the healing process. So eat plenty of citrus fruits or drink the juice.

But above all, eat in moderation. As we discussed in Chapter 1, a large belly can be a significant strain on the low back.

Q: Before we talk about exercise, what other lifestyle changes should I make?

A: While its precise role is a matter of debate, stress—as we discussed in Chapter 2—clearly is an important factor in back pain. It may be more easily said than done, but you should try to reduce the stress in your life.

There are a number of things you can do, from radical changes such as quitting a job in which you're stressed or unhappy, to such measures as psychotherapy, stress-management classes and self-help books—all of which may teach you basic coping mechanisms and relaxation techniques. And, of course, exercise can be a powerful means of eliminating or alleviating stress.

EXERCISE

Q: How helpful is exercise in preventing back problems?

A: It's generally considered one of the best things you can do for your back. In an article published in 1994 in the *Journal of the American Medical Association,* a group of University of Washington physicians, including Richard Deyo, reviewed 16 studies of the effect of exercise in preventing low-back pain, and found a statistically significant short-term benefit from exercise that strengthened back or abdominal muscles and improved overall fitness. People who exercised had fewer days of work lost because of back pain or fewer days of back pain, the researchers found.

Q: What kind of exercise is best for my back?

A: Exercise that makes the muscles in your back, stomach, hips and thighs strong and flexible. In that way, your spine not only gets support from the muscles that surround it, but relief from muscles elsewhere that help the back do its work.

For example, Lyle Micheli, M.D., an orthopedist at Harvard Medical School, says that a huge proportion of back problems stems from a lack of flexibility in major muscle groups in other parts of the body, like the hamstrings (which are in the backs of the thighs), quadriceps (in the fronts of the thighs), abdominals, and gluteals (in the buttocks). Athletes whose hamstrings are tight often get back pain, says Micheli, who pushes his patients to increase their flexibility until they can lift their legs to a 70- to 80-degree angle from the floor.

Q: Are there specific exercises for preventing back pain?

A: All of the exercises described in Chapter 2 for ailing backs also help in prevention. However, a prevention program for healthy backs includes exercises that work more muscles, more vigorously. Below, we list five exercises recommended by the American Academy of Orthopaedic Surgeons (AAOS).

- Wall slides to strengthen back, hip and leg muscles. Stand with your back against a wall and feet shoulder-width apart. Slide down into a crouch, with knees bent to about 90 degrees. Count to five and slide back up the wall.

- Leg raises to strengthen back and hip muscles. Lie on your stomach. Tighten the muscles in one leg and raise it from the floor. Hold your leg up for a count of 10 and return it to the floor. Do the same with the other leg.

- Leg raises to strengthen stomach and hip muscles. Lie on your back with your arms at your side. Lift one leg off the floor and hold it up for the count of 10. Return it to the floor and do the same with the other leg. (Alternatively, sit upright in a chair with your legs straight and raise each leg waist-high.)

- Partial sit-up to strengthen stomach muscles. Lie on your back with knees bent and feet flat on the floor. Slowly raise your head and shoulders off the floor and reach with both hands toward your knees.

• Back leg swing to strengthen hip and back muscles. Stand behind a chair with your hands on the back of the chair. Lift one leg back and up, while keeping the knee straight. Return slowly; raise the other leg and return.

All these exercises are to be done five times each. The AAOS recommends exercising every other day, limbering up first for a few minutes by moving your arms and legs and alternately tightening and relaxing your muscles. If you haven't exercised in some time, you can warm up by walking.

ERGONOMICS

Q: You said there are back-saving rules for everything. Let's start with my job—what should I do if I sit at a desk all day?

A: For starters, get a good chair. Different chairs have different uses, and the best chair for working at a computer, say, may not the best one for writing. Choose a chair that suits the activity you expect to do most.

In general, however, you should have good low-back support and be able to adjust your seat so your knees are slightly higher than your hips and your feet rest comfortably on the floor. If your feet are supported, not only will it reduce the stress on your low back, it will also inhibit you from twisting around to reach something in your office while you're sitting, which can strain your back.

If you're choosing the chair yourself, check for seat height, seat depth and width, seat tilt and cushion, backrest height, backrest support contour, seat-to-backrest angle, armrest height and distance between armrests. A chair may have up to 10 different controls to adjust these features to fit you.

Q: Sounds pretty expensive. How can I get my employer to pay for all that?

A: A 10-speed chair may be beyond your reach, but most ergonomic solutions are inexpensive, like raising or lowering the work surface, chair height or work product, according to John Triano, a chiropractor at the Texas Back Institute who was formerly director of the Spinal Ergonomics and Joint Research Laboratory at the National College of Chiropractic.

Many corrective measures can be homemade. If you can't adjust your seat, use a footrest or prop your feet on a box. If your chair doesn't support your lower back, tuck a pillow or a rolled-up towel behind your back.

Q: I sit at a computer all day. What else can I do to prevent back pain?

A: Watch your posture. That's critical for anybody who sits (or stands) all day, but it's particularly easy to fall into bad habits when you're glued to a monitor. Periodically change your posture throughout the day, which reduces the chance of back and neck pain. Also, adjust your monitor so the entire viewing area on the screen is somewhere below eye level. That will ensure your neck relaxes forward, rather than craning backward. Many offices invest in telephone headsets to prevent the "phone shoulder syndrome" described in Chapter 2.

Q: You've been talking mostly about sitting, but I have to stand for hours at a time—and my back hurts. What can I do?

A: According to back-care experts, you should try to maintain the natural curve of your spine. Keep one foot slightly higher than the other by resting it on a low stool, rail or platform. (That's why bars have bar rails!) Take turns, raising one foot, then the other.

Q: Okay, now I've got a chair and a footrest. What next?

A: Get out of your chair (or off your footrest) periodically to stretch your muscles. The publication *Body Bulletin* offers six stretches you can do at work:

While standing:

1. Bend both elbows. Press one above you and the other behind you for a good stretch.
2. Press your palms on your lower back for support. Gently arch your back, and hold for a moment.
3. To loosen stiff shoulders, circle them backward several times, then forward.
4. Press your elbows out and back at chest height as far as you can. Hold.

While sitting:

5. Sit back against a chair. Exhale and tighten your abdominal muscles for a count of 10.
6. Sit with your back and bottom pressed firmly against a hard, straight-backed chair. Lift your right arm

from the shoulder, reaching your fingertips toward the ceiling. Follow the movement with your neck and eyes. Hold for a few seconds and really feel that stretch. Repeat with left arm. Do each arm several times.

Q: Isn't my boss going to object if I start doing exercises?

A: Not if he or she knows what's good for business. According to Triano, "short, frequent breaks for highly repetitive job tasks will save more money in productivity than they will forfeit in work time lost." Triano says employers that have included a simple 10-minute program of stretching and flexibility exercises twice each day have reduced costs and increased worker morale and productivity.

Q: How much money are businesses saving by making ergonomic changes?

A: A number of companies have collected data showing substantial savings from such programs.

For example, at a Grumman Corporation plant employing 550 people, a three-year ergonomic safety program was credited with reducing back-injury costs to $36,832 in 1992, from $143,067 in 1990. Children's Hospital of San Diego, which implemented a customized back program because back injuries and costs soared in the early 1980s, found that its incidence of back injuries fell by more than half to 15 per 1,000 employees, and costs fell by $200,000 to $72,300.

Q: That's got to involve more than the way people sit. I suppose there are rules about the best way to lift heavy objects?

A: There certainly are. The American Academy of Orthopaedic Surgeons (AAOS) has launched a national public education program, "Lift It Safe," to teach people proper lifting methods and other ways to prevent back pain. It offers guidelines for lifting:

- Plan ahead what you want to do, and don't be in a hurry.

- Separate your feet shoulder-width apart to give you a solid base of support.

- Bend at the knees, *not* the waist; maintain the natural curve of your spine.

- Tighten your stomach muscles.

- Position the person or object close to your body before lifting.

- Lift with your legs.

- Avoid twisting your body; instead, point your toes in the direction you want to move and pivot in that direction.

- Do not try to lift an object that is too heavy or has an awkward shape. Get help.

For a free copy of the AAOS's "Lift It Safe" brochure, telephone (800) 824-BONE or send a stamped, self-addressed business-size envelope to Lift It Safe, American Academy of Orthopaedic Surgeons, P.O. Box 1998, Des Plaines, IL 60017.

Q: I drive all day. Do the same ergonomic rules apply to sitting in a car?

A: Yes and no. In both cases it's important to get breaks, so don't drive long distances without rest stops.

Ensuring a good seat will take more ingenuity. Use a low-back support, and two pillows under your passenger-side arm as an armrest if there isn't one in the car. Rest your other forearm on the armrest built into the door on the driver's side; if there isn't one, improvise.

Consider buying and using cruise control; it gives you more freedom to move about, shift your weight and change the position of your back. Tilt your rear view mirror up a bit. That forces you to sit up perfectly straight to see the cars behind you.

Finally, a tip Augustus White, a prominent orthopedist at Harvard Medical School, says he received from a patient: Don't carry your wallet in your back pocket if you have back pain and sciatica. The wallet presses on the sciatic nerve when you sit or drive, aggravating your condition.

SPORTS

Q: You said earlier that ergonomics has addressed recreational activities, too. What about sports?

A: A great many sports have been evaluated in terms of their impact—positive as well as negative—on the back. In fact, a number of sports are good for your back. To swimming and walking, which we recommended in Chapter 2, add bike riding and cross-country skiing. All of these can generally be done without sharp or sudden movements, hyperextension (severe arching) of the back, twisting or rotating the trunk, heavy impact and unexpected or awkward falls.

Q: But are there other sports I should avoid?

A: Many sports-medicine experts say no sport is intrinsically bad for your back, as long as it's practiced properly. Of course, the safety of any sport also depends on the type of back problem you have and the level of your conditioning.

Still, certain activities, like gymnastics, weight lifting, football and rowing, send up red flags for most orthopedists: Play at your peril. Other popular sports offer a moderate level of risk. Here's a list, with some precautions you can take to avoid injury:

- Running. Experts generally agree that running, particularly running fast, is hard on the back. If you must run, they say, do it every other day, run on soft surfaces and get the most impact-absorbent shoes you can find. If that doesn't help, says Harvard's White, switch to bicycling.

- Tennis. With its combination of vigorous twisting and turning, flexion and extension, tennis is considered a high-risk sport for people with back problems. Micheli advises players to flatten out their serves, thus eliminating excessive arching and twisting, and to consider wearing an elastic back brace to prevent extreme twists. Finally, doctors say, don't reach for every ball.

• Golf. In twisting violently to generate a powerful golf shot, players can damage discs and facet joints. To prevent this, White advises, smooth out the swing, twisting the back less and moving more at the hip and knee. And switch to nonspiked shoes or tennis shoes to reduce the impact at the end of the swing, and thus the irritation to your back.

Q: What do I need to condition myself for these sports?

A: Stay fit, use proper protective equipment and don't go to extremes. Many of the people who fill the waiting rooms of orthopedists and chiropractors are weekend athletes—people who are sedentary all week, yet throw themselves into a football game on Sunday.

Micheli, who is also director of the Division of Sports Medicine at Children's Hospital in Boston, advises people to develop their gluteal and quadriceps strength so they can crouch without excessively swaying the lower back. Younger athletes particularly need to follow a program of both stretching and strengthening, he says.

BACK SUPPORTS AND OTHER PRODUCTS

Q: What kinds of supports and other gear are good for my back?

A: Here's a partial list of some of the most common back aids:

• Backrests. Many back-care products are designed to reduce back pain and fatigue by encouraging good posture. One popular backrest consists of a contoured back with an attached seat. Some are inflatable, which is handy for airplane travel or other uses.

• Lumbar rolls. These are lightweight foam pillows that come in a variety of shapes—cylinders, curves—but are designed to be tucked behind your back when you sit in a chair.

• Neck supports. Stores and catalog houses sell "cervical pillows" that fit around the neck to keep it from rolling from side to side when you sleep. These can be useful for traveling in cars and planes.

For a discussion of braces, see Chapter 2.

Q: What about preventing whiplash? Do headrests on car seats work?

A: They can be very helpful if they're designed and positioned correctly—behind your head, not your neck. If your headrest is too low, and typically they are, adjust it or replace it with one that provides the necessary support.

Q: What about the back belts I see on men who do heavy lifting? Do those really work?

A: They get mixed reviews. A recent study by researchers in the orthopedics department at the University of California at San Diego found that so-called lumbar belts didn't help people lift more weight, and another study reported the belts didn't provide any protection against injury.

But you have to weigh that against the personal testimony of men like movers, who swear by them, and by certain ethnic people in Nepal, who for centuries have worn the *patuka,* a large piece of cloth wrapped around their waists, in the belief that it supports the low back and thus prevents back pain. Researchers who have investigated the use of the *patuka* by the famous Gurkha soldiers and others have concluded that it does reduce compression of the lumbosacral area.

How such belts help is as unclear as whether they help. It's been suggested that they work by reinforcing the extensor muscles, keeping those muscles warm, preventing overflexion, and serving as a constant reminder to lift properly.

Q: Are there any special tools designed for people with bad backs?

A: In addition to braces and other supports, there are a number of specially designed tools and furniture to help you garden, do office work and otherwise cope. Many of these are available from back-care specialty stores and catalog houses. Still other gear can be adapted for chores to reduce your risk:

- Yard work. There are lawn rakes and snow shovels with specially designed handles that take the strain off the back. Or you can just buy a lightweight model of a snow shovel with a plastic blade instead of a metal one.

• Housework. Because back-care experts advise getting down on one knee to avoid bending at the waist, you may want to protect your knees with sponge-rubber knee pads, available at any sports shop.

• Office work. Slant boards allow you to stand or sit erect, so you don't have to bend forward over a desk when you read or write. These boards, which have a bottom ledge on which books and papers rest upright, can be placed on a desk or even on a podium and adjusted to various angles.

• Grooming. Flexible two-foot-long shoehorns help you put on your shoes without bending your back much; so do loafers, as opposed to lace-up shoes.

Q: Any other advice about shoes?

A: As you probably suspected, high heels tend to shift the back into a slightly swaybacked position. However, a recent study showed that heels up to 1¾ inches don't increase or cause swayback. A safer but decidedly less glamorous bet is a flat shoe with a thick crepe or soft rubber sole and heel.

Q: What about mattresses?

A: Mattresses, like back products, come in an almost unimaginable variety—some of which are extremely helpful, others totally irrelevant. You won't get much guidance from the manufacturers, many of whom use terms like "posture," "osteopathic" and "orthopedic."

But research indicates that, as you've probably heard, firm is best. A study some 15 years ago, comparing the effects of four types of beds on patients with chronic low-back pain, found that most thought their backs improved after more than two weeks on a hard bed. A water bed came in second.

If you don't want to buy another mattress or risk sleeping on a sagging mattress when you're away from home, you might invest in a portable bed board that can be inserted between a mattress and box spring to provide firmness.

OTHER PREVENTIVE MEASURES

Q: Since we're on the subject of beds, let's talk about sex. Can't you throw your back out having sex?

A: When it comes to backs, "safe sex" does take on a whole new meaning. It's true that if you already have a problem back, sexual gymnastics and sexual marathons can certainly give you morning-after pain.

To prevent that, there are certain positions you should avoid—the standard missionary position, with its thrusting movements, is definitely one of them—and others you should try; the "spoon" position, in which both partners are on their sides with their hips and knees flexed, is one of those recommended. In general, positions in which the back is flexed, not extended, are safer.

If you have a problem back, don't be shy about asking your doctor or back-care provider for more specific information.

Q: My chiropractor said I should buy a "package" of weekly visits, even though my back stopped hurting. Is that a good idea?

A: That's a controversial subject, and one on which the expert panelists for the Rand study discussed in Chapter 2 were sharply divided. The chiropractors felt that people should continue maintenance manipulation after their symptoms have gone away, while the medical doctors felt there was no role for therapy once the pain was gone.

Q: Are there any studies proving that prevention actually works?

A: There are a number of studies, mainly about the effectiveness of exercise, which were reviewed in the *Journal of the American Medical Association* article mentioned earlier in this chapter. However, reviewers found the studies, most of which were conducted in the workplace, to be unimpressive. None followed up subjects beyond 18 months, and most combined people who had back problems with people who hadn't, so it was impossible to draw separate conclusions about the effectiveness of different strategies.

As a result, Deyo and his team said, the statistical evidence for prevention other than exercise—back schools, mechanical supports and modifying risk factors—was slim at best. There was "minimal" or "insufficient" evidence to confirm the use of either back belts or education programs about back mechanics. And none of the studies investigated what happened after people reduced smoking, lost weight or resolved psychological problems such as depression.

Q: Does that mean these measures aren't effective?

A: No. As Deyo's group noted, the studies didn't disprove the value of these strategies—they just didn't provide "statistically significant" support. The researchers did note there are plenty of "retrospective" studies—that is, studies carried out after the damage has been done—linking obesity and smoking to back problems.

In fact, there are a great many things you can do to prevent or alleviate back pain. Some are virtually certain to help; others may work for you. Doctors and others can help, but you can take charge. Back to you!

INFORMATIONAL AND MUTUAL-AID GROUPS

American Academy of Orthopaedic Surgeons
6300 N. River Rd.
Rosemont, IL 60018
(708) 823-7186 or (800) 346-2267

American Physical Therapy Association
1111 N. Fairfax St.
Alexandria, VA 22314
(703) 684-APTA

American Syringomyelia Alliance Project (ASAP)
(903) 236-7079 or (800) ASA-P282

Ankylosing Spondylitis Association
511 N. LaCienega Blvd.
Suite 216
Los Angeles, CA 90048
(310) 652-0609 or (800) 777-8189

Arthritis Foundation
1314 Spring St., N.W.
Atlanta, GA 30309
(800) 283-7800

Back Pain Association of America
P.O. Box 135
Pasadena, MD 21122
(410) 255-3633

International Chiropractors Association
1110 N. Glebe Rd.
Suite 1000
Arlington, VA 22201
(703) 528-5000

National Institute of Arthritis and Musculoskeletal and Skin Diseases
Information Clearinghouse
1 AMS Circle
31 Center Dr.
MSC2350
Bethesda, MD 20892-2350
(301) 495-4484

National Osteoporosis Foundation
1150 17th St., N.W.
Suite 500
Washington, DC 20036
(800) 223-9994

GLOSSARY

Acupuncture: An ancient Chinese healing art that involves inserting very thin needles into certain points along the body to relieve pain and promote healing.

Acute: Begins quickly and is intense or sharp; sharp or severe.

Allograph: Bone donated by one person and grafted onto another.

Ankylosing spondylitis: A type of arthritis, primarily affecting the spine and sacroiliac joints, in which bony bridges may form between vertebrae, causing the spine to become rigid.

Annulus: The tough outer fibrous portion of the intervertebral disc.

Arthritis: Inflammation and irritation of the joints.

Arthroscope: A flexible viewing tube containing optical fibers, a small lens and a light scope, that can be inserted into the disc to look directly at the material being removed.

Babinski reflex: A response to a physical exam that measures the condition of the spinal cord or brain.

Back school: An institution that teaches people how to go about their daily activities while protecting their backs. It provides instruction in the mechanics of the back and what causes back pain.

Bone densitometry: An X-ray technique that measures bone density.

Bone scan: A highly sensitive process that uses a radioactive substance to image the bone structure.

Cauda equina: The bundle of nerves in the spinal column, below the spinal cord, that controls the muscles of the legs, bladder, bowel and sexual function.

Cauda equina syndrome: A condition, generally requiring immediate surgery, in which massive disc herniation compresses the spinal cord or cauda equina.

Cervical spine: The neck or upper portion of the back, consisting of seven vertebrae which are enclosed by the rib cage.

Chemonucleolysis: A process in which chymopapain is injected into the intervertebral disc in order to break down its protein.

Chiropractic: A health-care practice that is based on the belief that the spinal column is central to well-being, and whose primary treatment is spinal manipulation or adjustment.

Chiropractor: A health-care practitioner who is awarded the degree of Doctor of Chiropractic (D.C.) after completing premedical studies followed by four years of training in an approved chiropractic school.

Chronic: Persisting for a long time.

Chymopapain: An enzyme that is sometimes injected into the nucleus of a bulging disc to reduce nerve compression.

Coccydynia: Pain in the coccyx, usually due to a hard fall or stress from prolonged sitting.

Coccyx: The structure, widely known as the tailbone, at the very tip of the spine.

Collagen: The fibrous tissue that supports and connects other tissues in the body.

Computerized axial tomographic scan (CT or **CAT scan):** A sophisticated X-ray imaging technique that produces cross-sectional images of body organs.

Cordotomy (or **Tractotomy):** A procedure dividing the spino-thalamic tract, which conducts pain from the body to the brain.

Corticosteroid: A steroid drug, related to the hormone cortisol, which may quickly reduce swelling and inflammation, but may have possible serious side effects.

Debridement: An operation in which an infected spine is cleaned, and pus, dead bone and foreign particles are washed out with antibiotics.

Decompression: The removal of pressure, typically from a herniated disc, on the nerves in the spinal canal.

Degenerative arthritis: See **Osteoarthritis.**

Disc: The flat, circular structure between vertebrae that acts as a shock absorber.

Disc degeneration: A condition, usually after the age of 30 or 40, in which discs gradually lose water, becoming less springy, smaller and less effective as shock absorbers.

Discectomy: The removal of all or part of the intervertebral disc.

Discitis: A painful inflammation of lumbar discs, believed to be caused by infection.

Discography: An imaging technique in which dye is injected into the center of the disc to show, through the way it leaks out, areas of herniation.

Electromyography (EMG): A method to test and record nerve and muscle function using electric impulses to stimulate the nerves.

Ergonomics: The scientific and clinical study of the healthiest use of the body in an occupational or recreational setting.

Erythrocyte sedimentation rate: A test that measures how fast red blood cells cling together, fall and settle to the bottom of a test tube. An elevated ''sed rate'' may indicate the presence of infection or inflammation.

Estrogen replacement therapy (ERT): A treatment often given older women to replace the estrogen lost as a result of menopause. When other hormones are added to estrogen, it is called hormone replacement therapy (HRT).

Extension: Backward bending of the spine.

Extensors (or **Erector spinae):** The back muscles responsible for extension and holding the spine erect.

Extrusion: A type of disc herniation in which the annulus ruptures but the containing ligament remains intact.

Facet joints: Paired joints, located behind the vertebral body, that connect the posterior elements of the vertebra.

Fascia: A specialized fibrous tissue that covers the muscle tissues of the back.

Fibrositis (or **Fibromyalgia** or **Myofascial pain):** A disease involving pain in muscles or joints with no clinical signs of inflammation.

Flexion: Forward bending of the spine.

Flexors: The muscles, including the abdominals, responsible for flexion.

Fluoridosis: A thickening of the bone, caused by excessive fluoride.

Foot drop: A condition, indicative of a ruptured disc pressing on a nerve, in which people drag their feet because their leg muscles cannot raise their toes.

Foramen: An opening in a membrane or bone.

Free fragments: Nuclear material from the herniated disc that is floating freely in the spinal canal or at the nerve exits.

Fusion: See **Spinal fusion.**

Gold salts: Gold compounds, given by injection or orally, to treat rheumatoid arthritis.

Herniated disc (or **Ruptured disc**)**:** Displacement of part of the disc's soft center beyond the normal confines of the annulus.

Hyperlordosis: Excess lordosis or swayback.

Ibuprofen: A nonsteroidal anti-inflammatory agent.

Idiopathic: In medical language, refers to the lack of known origin.

Inflammation: The body's protective response to an injury or infection.

Kinesiotherapist: A health-care professional specializing in long-term rehabilitation.

Kyphosis: The normal, slight backward curve of the thoracic spine.

Lamina: The bony plate on the back of the vertebrae.

Laminectomy: The surgical procedure in which the entire lamina at a certain level is removed to permit access to the spinal canal.

Laminotomy: A procedure similar to the laminectomy, but with only partial removal of the lamina.

Ligaments: Rubbery bands of strong fibrous tissue that bind bones or other body parts together, keeping them in alignment.

Lordosis: The natural forward curve of the lumbar spine, when viewed from the side.

Lumbar spine: The low back, consisting of five vertebrae.

Magnetic resonance imaging (MRI): An imaging technique that can produce pictures of soft tissues that would not be seen on an X-ray.

Massage: Working on the soft tissue, kneading muscle to reduce stiffness and pain and increase circulation.

Meningioma: A benign tumor that occurs in the thoracic spine or spinal canal.

Meningitis: Any infection or swelling of the membranes covering the brain and spinal cord.

Microdiscectomy: A discectomy performed through an operating microscope, allowing a smaller incision and a less invasive procedure.

Multiple myelomas: Malignant tumors of the bone marrow that may originate in the spine.

Myelography: Injection of a dye or contrast material into the spinal canal that, through imaging, allows evaluation of the spinal canal and nerve roots.

Neurofibroma: Malignant tumor of the spine that begins in the nerve roots.

Neurologist: A physician specializing in the brain, spinal cord and peripheral nerves.

Neurosurgeon: A physician who performs surgery in areas of neurological interest.

Nonsteroidal anti-inflammatory drugs (NSAIDs): A group of drugs, including aspirin, ibuprofen and many prescription drugs, having pain-relieving, fever-reducing and anti-inflammatory effects.

Occupational therapist: A health-care professional who provides services designed to restore self-care, work and leisure skills of people who have specific performance incapacities.

Orthopedist (or **Orthopedic surgeon):** A physician who specializes in treatment and surgery of the joints and related structures.

Osteoarthritis: Degenerative arthritis of both the disc and the facet joints, frequently caused by old age or joint injury.

Osteoclasts: The body's bone-destroying cells.

Osteoid osteoma: A bony tumor that, although benign, can cause severe back pain.

Osteopath: A physician whose training, in addition to the usual techniques of drugs, surgery and radiation, has emphasized the musculoskeletal system.

Osteophyte (or **Bone spur**)**:** A bony growth around the joints, seen in people with osteoarthritis. Joints may appear to be swollen.

Osteoporosis: A condition, prevalent in the elderly, in which bones lose density and strength, and are more susceptible to fracture.

Osteotomy: Radical surgery, involving fracturing the spine and removing a wedge of bone, to treat ankylosing spondylitis.

Paget's disease of the bone: A disorder, often associated with osteoarthritis, in which the bones may weaken and fracture easily.

Percutaneous discectomy: A procedure in which part of the herniated disc is removed with suction.

Physiatrist: A physician specializing in noninvasive treatment such as physical therapy, rehabilitation and lifestyle changes.

Physical therapist: A health-care professional who is licensed to assist in testing and treating physically disabled persons.

Physical therapy: Treatment emphasizing exercise, heat and cold, and massage.

Prolapse (or **Protrusion**)**:** A distension of the intervertebral disc with containment of the nucleus within the stretched annulus.

Prosthesis: The artificial replacement of a body part.

Pseudarthrosis: A situation in which spinal fusion fails, leaving the back painful and unstable.

Psoas: Muscles, beginning at the front of the lumbar spine, whose main job is to move the legs.

Psychosocial: Factors such as stress, depression and satisfaction with one's work and/or life, which can influence the advent or course of back pain.

Radiculopathy: Radiating pain in the arms or legs caused by a pinched nerve.

Reiter's syndrome: A condition whose symptoms include spinal arthritis, low-back pain, and inflammation of the urethra and of the eye or other mucous membrane.

Rheumatoid arthritis: A chronic disease with inflammatory changes occurring through the body's connective tissues.

Rheumatologist: A doctor who specializes in the treatment of arthritis, especially rheumatoid arthritis and other inflammatory diseases.

Rhizotomy (or **Rhizolysis**): A pain-relieving surgical procedure in which the nerves around facet joints are destroyed.

Sacroiliac: The joint where the sacrum meets the pelvis on each side.

Sacrum: The triangular bone consisting of five vertebrae fused together, immediately below the lumbar spine.

Schwannoma: One type of malignant tumor of the spine.

Sciatic nerve: A long nerve stretching through the muscles of the thigh, leg and foot, with many branches.

Sciatica: A condition, generally caused by a herniated disc, in which there is pain in the body supplied by the sciatic nerve—that is, the buttock, thigh and leg.

Scoliosis: An abnormal curvature of the spine.

Sequestration: A complete herniation of the disc material through the annulus and supporting posterior ligament.

Somatic: Relating to the body rather than to the mind.

Spasm: Intensely contracted, painful muscles, either alternating or persistent.

Spinal canal: The cavity within the vertebral column through which the spinal cord runs.

Spinal column (or **Spine**)**:** The entire group of 24 vertebrae which connect to the skull and end with the coccyx.

Spinal cord: The extension of the brain, through which nerves travel, ending at the top of the lumbar spine.

Spinal fusion: A procedure in which two or more vertebrae are connected with a bone graft to reduce motion and eliminate pain.

Spinal manipulation: The practice, most closely identified with chiropractic, of applying pressure to the spine to restore alignment and mobility.

Spinal stenosis: A degenerative condition in which the spinal column narrows and encroaches upon the spinal canal, pressing on the nerves that run through it.

Spinous processes: Knob-like projections from the vertebrae that form an extra protective wrapping around the spinal canal.

Spondylitis: A swelling of any of the spinal vertebrae, usually marked by stiffness and pain.

Spondylolisthesis: A condition in which, due to a defect or crack, vertebrae tend to slip out of alignment.

Spondylolysis: An anatomic gap in the back of a vertebrae, due to defects or cracks.

Spondylolytic: See **Spondylolisthesis** and **Spondylolysis.**

Sprain: Tear in the muscle or ligament.

Strain: Overstretching of the muscle or ligament.

Subluxation: A partial dislocation in the normal position of two adjacent vertebrae. Orthopedists believe this should be visible through imaging, chiropractors do not.

Synovial: Descriptive of the tissue lining the facet joints that secrete a lubricating fluid.

Syringomyelia: A painful condition caused when cysts form in the spinal canal and press against nerves.

Thoracic spine: The midback, consisting of 12 vertebrae enclosed by the rib cage.

Thoracotomy: A complex surgical procedure on the middle back or thorax to reach a herniated thoracic disc.

Traction: A force applied along the axis of the spine in an attempt to elongate it and thus allow nerve decompression.

Transcutaneous electrical nerve stimulation (TENS): A treatment that involves administering pulses of low-voltage electric current to the back.

Vertebrae: The 24 bones that comprise the spine.

Vertebral osteomyelitis: Probably the most common spinal infection, affecting the vertebral body.

Video-assisted thoracoscopy (VAT): Thoracic spine surgery performed with the use of fiber optics and video imaging.

Whiplash: A partial dislocation of the cervical vertebral facet joints, resulting in injury to the adjacent soft tissue.

SUGGESTED READING

Abraham, Edward A. *Freedom From Back Pain: An Orthopedist's Self-Help Guide.* Emmaus, Penn.: Rodale Press, 1986.

The American Medical Association Book of Back Care. New York: Random House, 1982.

The Back Almanac. Oakland, Calif.: Lanier, 1992.

Bonati, Alfred O., and Shirley Linde. *No More Back Pain.* New York: Scripps Howard, 1991.

Fraser, Richard, and Ann Forer. *The Well-Informed Patient's Guide to Back Surgery.* New York: Dell, 1992.

Hall, Hamilton. *More Advice From the Back Doctor.* Toronto: McClelland and Stewart, 1987.

Hochschuler, Stephen. *Back in Shape.* Boston: Houghton Mifflin, 1991.

Klein, Arthur C., and Dava Sobel. *Backache Relief.* New York: Times Books, 1985.

McIlwain, Harris H., et al. *Winning With Back Pain.* New York: John Wiley & Sons, 1994.

Swezey, Robert L., and Annette M. Swezey. *Good News for Bad Backs.* New York: Knightsbridge, 1990.

White, Augustus A., III. *Your Aching Back: A Doctor's Guide to Relief.* New York: Simon and Schuster/Fireside, 1990.

YMCA Healthy Back Book. Champaign, Ill: Human Kinetics Publishers, 1994.

INDEX

A

B

C

D

E

F

G

H

I

K

L

M

N

O

P

R

S

T

U

V

W

X

Y